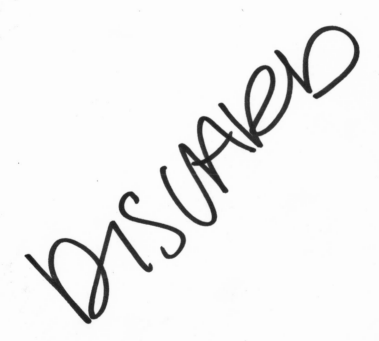

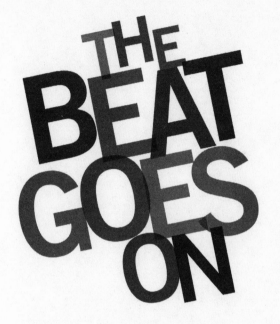

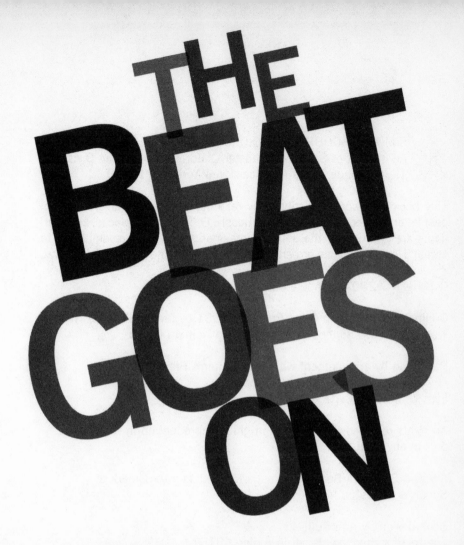

THE BEAT GOES ON

ADELE MINCHIN

SIMON & SCHUSTER BOOKS FOR YOUNG READERS
New York   London   Toronto   Sydney

SIMON & SCHUSTER BOOKS FOR YOUNG READERS
An imprint of Simon & Schuster Children's Publishing Division
1230 Avenue of the Americas, New York, NY 10020

Originally published in Great Britain in 2001 by Livewire Books, The Women's Press Limited, a member of the Namara Group

Published by arrangement with The Women's Press Ltd.

First U.S. edition, 2004

Book design by Ann Sullivan
The text for this book is set in Aldine 401BT.

Manufactured in the United States of America
10 9 8 7 6 5

CIP data for this book is available from the Library of Congress.
0-689-86611-9

For all the young people who
continue the brave struggle

THE BEAT GOES ON

ONE

I'D BEEN STARING AT THE SAME WALLS IN THE POKY box bedroom of our semidetached house since I emerged into this world kicking and screaming fifteen years ago. I was lying star-shaped on my double bed, tuning into the same noises of the same Saturday night routine that I'd been tuning into since I was in my playpen. The walls of our house are so thin I can hear our neighbors' every move. Sometimes I think I can hear them breathing. Mr. Davies from next door has been padding up the stairs to the back bedroom of his house, opening the bedside table drawer, pulling out his pipe, and then slamming the bedroom door behind him every Saturday night for as long as I can remember. It's his Saturday night treat to go outside and smoke his pipe while surveying his garden. Come hail, rain, or snow, he's out there without fail. I always lie still until he's gone and then peep over my windowsill to check that he's in the garden and out of earshot so that I can start breathing again. I can't bear to think of him having an ear on my world as well.

Sadie, my older sister, was getting ready in her room next to mine. I could hear her emptying her makeup bag onto her bed to choose her lipstick and eye shadow. She was going to the Bull and Gate with her boyfriend, Anthony. They've been going there every Saturday night for the past five years, ever since they started going out with each other. They never go anywhere out of Bury together apart from their annual fortnight's holiday in the sun. No sooner have they come back from one trip—the wheels of the plane have barely had time to hit the runway—before they've booked the same two weeks' holiday in Minorca for the following year. Sadie has worked at the building society, Abbey National (or Grabby National, as my dad calls it), since she left school four years ago. All she does is moan about her job, but she never does anything to change her situation. She says she doesn't know what else to do. Anthony is a policeman. They're so boring I practically fall into a coma just thinking about them.

Mum and Dad were sitting downstairs in our white-with-a-hint-of-apple lounge, surrounded by Mum's prized knickknacks. Mum is so house-proud she borders on compulsive-obsessive. She gets all of her "better home" ideas from daytime TV and is dead proud of herself for being all creative when she turns an old table into an elegant piece of furniture by throwing a peach bedsheet over it and plonking a vase of dried flowers on top. She's just got into stenciling as well. Every blank piece of wall in our house has undergone the stencil treatment. No single sheet of wallpaper is safe from my mum's paintbrush or the free stenciling kit that came stuck to the front of *Good Housekeeping*. If you stand still for too long you find yourself with a recurring flower-and-leaf motif stenciled to your forehead.

Mum was watching *Who Wants to Be a Millionaire*. I could hear her getting more and more frustrated with the contestants and screaming her answers at the screen. Dad was asleep in the armchair with the *Daily Mail*'s sports section spread out over his lap.

I knew it was eight thirty because Sadie had just popped her head round the lounge door to tell Mum and Dad that she was going down the Bull and Gate with Anthony. As if they didn't already know. You'd have thought she'd have realized that they can predict where she's off to without her having to announce it each week like it's something new. Dad woke up from his snooze and him and Mum both chorused, "Have a nice time." It's like an alarm clock telling me to get out and do something less boring instead. I wish that one Saturday Mum would turn round to Sadie and say, "Yes dear, and your dad and I are off to a salsa bar in town and then we're going to nosh down a curry in Rusholme before heading off to an all-night rave. See you in the morning."

But after what I found out that Saturday I was more aware than ever of the cozy routine of our household. It's amazing how much you take for granted in this life. I used to take everything for granted—my mum's neurotic little routines, our house, my monthly allowance, my education, my health, my mum and dad, my stupid sister and her nightmare boyfriend. They were just there. I used to wake up in the morning and everything was exactly as I'd left it the night before and the night before that and the night before that. I'm sure it's the same for almost everyone. But that day it suddenly wasn't the same.

Imagine if one day you woke up and circumstances had changed so dramatically that your entire world had been turned completely upside down and you couldn't take anything for granted anymore. I found out that life can have a very funny way of creeping up on you from behind and taking you by surprise just when you're least expecting it. After living in this household for fifteen years, where everything has been operating on a strict timetable since the beginning of time, I didn't think surprise or anything out of the ordinary was possible. I'd always prayed for change in my life. I'd always wanted something exciting to happen, to banish the routine and mundane reality of it all forever. But I hadn't expected this to happen. God, I'd have done anything for this not to have happened. I never wanted *this*.

Perhaps the messages I'd been sending out into the cosmos while lying star-shaped on my bed begging for something exciting and unpredictable to happen had been taken down incorrectly; maybe somebody had got it all wrong.

I'd written a cosmic shopping list at the beginning of the year as part of my New Year's resolutions. I'd read all about it in some magazine and it said that if you write down exactly what you want, hide it away somewhere special, and believe in it enough, your wishes will come true eventually. Number four on my cosmic shopping list was: "I want a good drama in my life." Well, that wish definitely came true. Something dramatic did happen, and nothing will ever be the same again. But it wasn't *supposed* to be like this.

It drove me mad watching and listening to everything carry on as normal all around me when so much had changed. But I couldn't tell a soul. Emma had made me promise not to tell a living being.

Emma is my cousin. She lives in a flat above the chemist in town with Aunty Jean, my mum's sister. Her dad left when she was only seven. Aunty Jean found a love letter from another woman hidden in one of his jackets and she went ballistic. She took the letter to work and got it enlarged and photocopied a hundred times. Then she bought some wallpaper paste and papered the whole of their kitchen with the love letter. Uncle Kevin came home from work that day and found the evidence of his affair plastered all over the kitchen. I wish I could have seen his face; he must have had the shock of his life. He packed his bags and left that very same night, and they haven't heard from him since. Aunty Jean was devastated. She went a bit funny for a while but she's all right now.

She and Mum aren't very close—they're too different and just don't get on. Mum is quiet and conservative and likes to keep herself to herself. Aunty Jean thinks my mum's a snob. Sometimes I wish me and Sadie were close, but we're just too different as well. Sadie looks at me like I'm from another planet most of the time. I'm closer to Emma really. She's only a year older than me and feels more like a sister to me. She understands me better, and we like the same things.

Emma goes to a sixth-form college in Manchester. She used to go to the convent in Bury, but she wanted to do Spanish A Level and she changed to the college because it's on the curriculum there. She's mad about traveling, and reckons that by learning languages she's equipping herself with all the ammunition she needs to get out of Bury and off to more exciting destinations. A bunch of her mates from the convent have gone to the same college, so she's not on her own, but she seems to have settled in with everyone else there as well. I'm sure she'll be as popular as ever.

She's dead pretty, with this gorgeous natural curly blond hair that she cuts really short. The tight curls frame her heart-shaped face and show off her startling blue eyes. She's got a little scar just above her right eyebrow where she used to have a piercing until it went septic, so she's just got her nose pierced now, with a blue diamond stud that shows off the blue of her eyes. She's tall and slim and wears hipster jeans effortlessly, plus skinny-rib T-shirts with logos on like GLAMOUR IS MY PROFESSION. If Emma was a flower she'd be a sunflower—tall and strong, radiating light and energy. If I was a flower I'd be your average daffodil—nice enough but nothing special, not the sort of flower that people stop and admire. I've got mousy brown hair to my shoulders with a severe fringe that I cut myself. If I had to choose the thing I like most about myself it would be my tummy. It's round and comforting and always seems to stay brown from sunbathing in the summer much longer than the rest of my body. Emma convinced me to get my belly button pierced at the same time she got her eyebrow done, so I like wearing short tops that show it off. Apart from that I look pretty average, especially next to Em.

Emma is a real happy-go-lucky kind of person. She's just naturally contented. She's always telling me off for thinking too much and says I should enjoy the moment more. She's one of those people who is really free and easy and doesn't lack any confidence whatsoever. If you look up the word "relaxed" in the dictionary, there's a photo of Emma smiling back at you with her great big cheesy grin.

We always have a laugh, whatever we do together. She's always mad for getting up to some sort of mischief.

I remember one year the fair came to town—we must have been about twelve or thirteen at the time—and she decided that she was going to leave school to go and work at the fair. She said she was born to live a nomadic lifestyle where each day brought something new. She bunked off school and managed to convince the manager of the fair to let her work on the waltzers for the day to prove how hardworking and serious she was about joining the team. She told him she was sixteen. I was downtown with my best friend Sarah after school and we saw Em stood in the middle of the waltzers, sleeves rolled up above her elbows, pushing the cars around with all her might. Sarah and I leapt on and had the ride of our lives. Em started twirling us round as though we were just feathers in the wind. The more we screamed at her to stop pushing us so hard, the faster she'd push, until Sarah was sick all over her shoes and I was nearly sick from laughing so much. Dave, the manager, said she was the best worker he'd ever seen and offered her a six-month contract.

But her career in the fair didn't last long, because her mum caught her on her way home from work and dragged her off home—not, however, before challenging Emma to a competition on the Dodgem cars first. Aunty Jean said it would do them both good to vent their frustrations bashing around in some old cars before they went home and she gave Emma the telling-off of a lifetime.

It was funny to think of them being so easygoing with each other after what'd happened. I knew something was wrong when I bumped into Emma and Aunty Jean coming out of the doctor's the week before. They weren't their usual selves. Emma looked as though she'd been crying. Her nose was red and her usually immaculate mascara and eyeliner were smudged halfway down her face. She wouldn't look me in the eye, and instead tucked herself in close beside Aunty

Jean, huddling for protection. It was as though she just wanted to disappear. It wasn't like Emma at all. Aunty Jean said Emma had just got a bad dose of the flu and they were worried it was glandular fever because there was so much of it going around, so they'd popped to the doctor's for a checkup. Her face looked strained and her eyes were red, but she chatted cheerily nonetheless.

"They say it's a kissing disease, and you know what Emma's like for kissing the lads," Aunty Jean said with a smile, nudging Emma in the ribs. Emma flashed her a look of hurt and anger and seemed to be on the brink of tears. She flung herself away and stormed off to the other side of the road. Aunty Jean rushed over to put her arm around her, which Em rejected forcefully. I couldn't understand why she was acting so moodily and I teased her for being such a baby. Aunty Jean was visibly upset and was backpedaling madly to try to console her. I could hear her saying that she hadn't meant what she'd said and that she wasn't thinking straight. It wasn't like Em to be so sensitive. "She's just run-down—you know what it's like when you've got flu. Best get her straight to bed, I reckon. Send my love to your mum. Tell her to come and see us some-time if she can get down off her throne," Aunty Jean said.

So they'd headed off through the drizzle in the direction of their flat, huddled tightly together, heads bent low as if shielding themselves from more than just the rain.

That night I'd walked home puzzling over what on earth had got into Emma. She'd acted so strangely. I'd seen her be offhand with her mum before, but nothing like she was out-side the doctor's. I'd always wanted to tell her how lucky she was to have a mum like hers who would do anything for her and was always such good fun.

I can remember being so lost in thought over Emma's bizarre behavior—well, and the new songbook I'd bought before I bumped into her—that I forgot to buy the bread and milk Mum had asked me to get on my way back from school. I'd hoped to go straight to our garage where my drum kit is kept, and have time for a good bash around before tea, but I knew there would be hell to pay for forgetting the bread and milk. Mum just doesn't give me a break. If she's not giving me grief for being slovenly and selfish, she's threatening to call the police to report me for noise pollution for playing my drums "too loud, too late." I've got a curfew of eight o'clock and if I run overtime she comes sweeping into the garage wagging her finger and telling me to wind it up.

That night me and Mum rowed again, as usual. "I can't trust you to do anything for me," Mum said, shaking her head over her cup of black tea. "Me, me, me—that's all you think about. I bet you were swanning around that music shop not giving your family a second thought."

"I bumped into Aunty Jean and Em coming out of the doctor's. Em's ill. Aunty Jean was upset and was taking Em home to wait on her hand and foot. Fat chance of getting any of that treatment round here," I added under my breath.

"I beg your pardon?" Nothing slips past my mother. "Jean spoils that girl rotten. Ever since Kevin walked out on them she's given her everything, and it's just not good for her. She doesn't learn any discipline. So enough of your cheek, madam, and be glad you've got a mother who cares about you enough to bring you up properly." Mum's grip tightened around her mug and a frown deepened along her brow as I lost her to deep, dark thoughts of a family gone wrong.

I couldn't be bothered to argue with her. I'd heard the

same old things so many times before. Yawn, yawn. Stick another record on, Mum. I didn't want to waste any more time listening to her trying to settle old accounts with her sister. All I could think about was drowning out all the boring family history by playing my drums as loud as I could. As I skulked off to the garage without Mum even noticing, I breathed a sigh of relief.

TWO

IT WAS EARLY ON SATURDAY MORNING THAT I'D BEEN woken by a strange tapping at my bedroom window. It had filtered into my dreams, and I'd ignored it for a while, until the noise got louder and louder and I thought the glass was going to come crashing in. I threw off the duvet and stomped grumpily to the window, only to find Emma stood in our back garden, clutching a handful of grit and stones, beckoning me to come down. I flung the window open to ask her what exactly she was doing there at eight o'clock on a Saturday morning and why she couldn't use the doorbell like everyone else.

"Sshh! Be quiet or you'll wake your parents up. Just get dressed and meet me at the end of the road."

I was so curious to find out what she was up to that I got dressed in a flash and was out of the door and down the road before Mum had time to twitch at her net curtains.

Em was leaning against the lamppost at the end of my road, staring at her feet and pulling on a loose thread in her cardigan. She didn't even notice me in front of her.

"Cooee! Helloww! You woke me up, remember?"

She looked up slowly and managed a faint smile. I noticed that she had huge black rings under her eyes; she looked as though she'd been crying again. I'd spoken to her a couple of days after I'd bumped into her outside the doctor's, and I knew that she'd recovered from the flu after a lot of pampering from her mum, so something else had to be wrong.

"Hey, are you okay, Em? You don't look too hot. Huh, I guess I can't talk. But then again *I* was rudely awakened."

"Yeah, sorry about that. I, umm . . . I, uhh . . . just need to talk to you about something, that's all, and couldn't face seeing your mum and dad."

"I know how you feel—I can't *ever* face seeing them. So what's up?"

"Where shall we go? Is there somewhere round here we can talk without being heard?"

"Weyhey, gossip and scandal first thing on a Saturday morning. Fantastic," I said, rubbing my hands together in anticipation.

"No, seriously, Leyla, where can we go?"

"Well, it is eight A.M., you know. There's not going to be that many people around at this time of the morning. We can go down to the lake."

There's a park near my housing estate where I always go to be alone and to get away from Mum and Dad, so we went and sat down by the lake there. On our way Emma told me that she had something really important to say and that she was only telling me because she knew that she could trust me. Before she told me anything, however, I had to vow not to tell a soul. She pulled out a crinkled picture of her and Aunty Jean together at the beach in Scarborough last year and asked me to put my hand over the photo and swear on their lives that I wouldn't tell anybody what she was about to tell me. She said that their lives depended on my being loyal to them. It sounded pretty serious, but by this time I was bursting to know what she had to say. I love gossip, and from the buildup that Emma was giving this particular piece of news I was sure it was going to be juicy. But something in Emma's eyes and her distant manner made me slow down and hide my excitement at the prospect of this important news.

Emma was paranoid that someone would hear us talking, and she wouldn't open her mouth until she was satisfied that we were completely alone. She stared into space a lot, threw stones into the lake, and kept scuffing up her shoes in the mud. I bit my lip and chewed on my newly grown fingernails, trying to be patient and let her tell me in her own time whatever it was she had to say.

We sat in silence for quite a while, but eventually I just had to give her a nudge. We'd been staring into space for so long I wasn't sure if she was still breathing.

"Earth calling Miss Stevens. Emma, what is it? What's happened?" I searched her eyes for a hint of what she could possibly have to tell me.

She still didn't say anything for a long time. One minute she looked as though she was just about to open her mouth and say something, but then she'd start fidgeting around, ripping at the grass and digging her nails into the soil.

"Have you heard from your dad or something? Is it

something to do with your mum? Em, what's up? Come on, tell me what's going on."

"I just don't know how to say the words. I'm so confused. I'm so . . . Oh God, I just can't believe what's happening to me."

"Emma, please tell me. You're scaring me now. Just take a deep breath and let it all out."

"Oh Leyla, *I'm* scared as well. I'm terrified. There's something wrong with me. Something terrible has happened, and to be honest I can't quite believe it's true. I've been to the doctor's. I've had some tests. I've been so frightened."

Then it suddenly dawned on me. She was pregnant. Of course. No wonder she was acting so strangely and wanted so much privacy before she told me. That's why she'd been to the doctor's last week and why, when I'd seen her outside, she was so weepy and defensive. My heart sank.

"You're pregnant, aren't you," I said, reaching out for her hand.

"Oh, I wish, Leyla, I wish. That would be so simple." She snatched her hand away.

"What are you talking about? What's wrong with you? What's happened? What did the doctor say?" I was shocked.

"Leyla, you have to promise not to tell anyone. I mean *anyone*. This is the hardest thing I've ever had to do in all my life. It's so awful I just don't know how to say it." She took a big deep breath, turned to face me, looked at me square in the eyes for the first time all morning, and said, "Leyla, I'm . . . I'm . . . I'm HIV positive."

I giggled nervously and punched her playfully in the arm. "What do you mean?" I looked at her, desperately trying to understand what she was telling me. It was as though I couldn't understand English anymore.

"Leyla, I'm HIV positive. You know, AIDS? All that stuff about a disease you can get if you don't have safe sex? Well, it's actually happened to me." Emma burst into tears, flinging her head into her hands.

"Oh my God." I clamped my hand to my mouth. My stomach turned over and I felt sick and dizzy all of a sudden. I looked at her crying, writhing in her personal agony, and replayed her words in my head over and over again: "I'm HIV positive. I'm HIV positive." Out loud, I muttered, "Oh my God. Oh my God. Emma, Emma. Oh, Emma. I just . . . I can't believe it."

I don't know how long I sat there with my hand over my mouth, gasping and shaking from head to toe, but it felt like an eternity. When I finally pulled myself together I drew Emma to me and hugged her and held her as tight as I could. She sobbed uncontrollably in my arms and we held each other and cried for a very long time, silent apart from our snuffling and snivels.

Eventually Emma pulled herself away. She sat bolt upright and stared straight ahead. She suddenly seemed so distant, so far away from me. The shock and distress, the sheer gravity of everything she had just told me created a yawning gulf between us. She was sat right next to me, but we were a million miles apart. It was the distance that frightened me the most. I wanted to draw her close, tell her everything would be okay, wipe her tears and soothe the pain away. But we both knew that no sticking plaster or sweet cup of tea was going to make this all better. I didn't know what to say or do. I felt completely helpless and stupid as I just sat there, unable to say anything or help her in any way.

After an age of silence, Emma spoke. "You must be

wondering how and why," she said, still looking straight ahead, her face blank and expressionless.

"I'm just so . . . shocked. It's such a shock. I mean, are you ill *now*? Are you in pain?"

"No, I'm not in pain. I'm not even ill. I haven't got so much as a cold. Funny, huh? I've been told I've got this dreadful disease and I've never felt better in all my life. It's funny, isn't it?" She was laughing, tears pouring down her face.

Staring into her grief-soaked face, I was struck by a moment of clarity. They'd got her test results mixed up with someone else's. It was always happening. Emma couldn't have HIV. It just wasn't possible. They'd obviously made a mistake.

"Em, are you sure they've got it right? They could be wrong, you know. I saw this story on the news the other day about this woman who'd been told that she had breast cancer. She had one of her breasts removed to stop the cancer from spreading and then they found out that she'd been given the wrong results and she didn't have cancer at all. You're always hearing stories like that. They could be wrong. I reckon you should get a second opinion. They're probably wrong."

"Leyla, I had the test done almost four months ago. I've been to and from the clinic talking to experts and counselors about it for weeks. They haven't made a mistake. It was me who made the mistake: sleeping with someone without using a bloody condom."

"You mean you've known about this for four months and you haven't told anyone?"

"I told my mum."

"Oh my God. Your mum knows? She must have had a heart attack."

"Apparently some people don't tell anyone for years that

they've got it. I just had to tell my mum, though. After I'd got my results from the clinic I had some counseling and they asked me if there was anyone I could talk to because I shouldn't go through it on my own. Mum was the only person I wanted to run to, but I was terrified of telling her. I didn't know how she'd handle it. I thought she'd be so disgusted with me, she'd throw me out or something. I'm so ashamed of what's happened. I feel as though it's all my fault and that I deserve to be abandoned, but I had to tell her. I gave my consent for the woman at the clinic to call her, but they encouraged me to tell her myself when she arrived. They said it would be better if I spoke the words and spelt it out to her, rather than watching them tell her. They wanted me to take control of the situation, which was good, looking back on it now, because I felt as though I was watching my life spiral out of control before my eyes.

"She came down and I told her there and then, only a few hours after I'd been given the results. If I hadn't done it then I don't think I ever would have. I would have been too scared to even leave the clinic and go home, the state I was in. We were in this room with the counselor for hours, just sobbing our hearts out. Mum couldn't stop crying after the shock of it had sunk in. It was a good job we got it all out in the open there because at least she had professionals she could bombard with questions and get expert answers from." Emma was talking quickly, rambling through her explanation of events, barely stopping for air. I got the feeling she was trying to avoid any silences and drown out the shock of the news.

"You should have told me sooner."

"How could I? I've been so scared. I didn't know how anyone would react. I'm so scared of being on my own, of everyone abandoning me. I didn't even believe it myself for ages. Just like you, I kept thinking that they must have got it wrong."

"So how come you're telling me now?"

"I'm going mad keeping this dark, horrible secret from everyone. Everyone's noticing a difference in me, but I can't tell a soul what's really wrong. Mum and the counselor said that it might help to talk to a close friend my age whom I could trust. I told them I wanted to tell you and they suggested I do it at the clinic, with professionals around to help me, but I decided that I wanted to do it on my own. I can talk to Lucia and Jo about most stuff. I mean, they've been my best mates all the way through school and we know everything about one another, but this is different. This has got so many implications and consequences I just don't know if they could handle it or whether, at the moment, I could handle telling them. It would be so hard for them to keep such a huge secret. At least with you I know that if I ask you not to tell anyone then you're not going to. Maybe in time I'll tell them. Who knows?"

"Oh, Em, I'm so shocked. I just don't know what to say. I'm not even sure I know what HIV is exactly. I mean, have you got AIDS as well or what? It doesn't mean you're going to die, does it?" I could feel the panic rise to my throat, preventing me from breathing properly.

"HIV is the virus that causes AIDS. Believe me, I know everything there is to know about it all. I've been to that clinic so many times."

"So what does that mean then? You can have HIV and not AIDS?"

"HIV is the virus that attacks the immune system so your body can't fight off infections. As a result you can go on to develop certain serious illnesses and that's when they call it AIDS." Emma broke off. "Listen to me. I sound like a friggin' doctor."

I felt her drifting away from me again. I knew she was wondering what I was thinking, but at that point I just didn't know what to think or say. My mind was blank with shock. Emma stared out over the lake and licked tears from the corner of her mouth. Rain began to fall quite heavily, plastering my hair to my head, which seemed to weigh my brain down even more. Neither of us moved. My mind was racing, but nothing would come out of my mouth. I was so frightened of saying the wrong thing I felt as though I'd lost the ability to speak.

I watched the rain make patterns in the surface of the lake, and this seemed to hypnotize me, slow me down. I thought how it always seemed to be raining lately. Everything was damp. Our classrooms at school had that lingering fusty smell of damp about them. Mum was always complaining that our clothes were taking forever to dry.

I suddenly panicked that I hadn't put a sheet over my drum kit to protect it from damp in the garage at home. I almost voiced my panic out loud, but when I turned around to Emma I realized that I'd let my mind wander. Seeing her, sodden from tears and rain, I felt the urge to pick her up and carry her to a safe, warm, dry place and look after her forever. I placed my hand in hers and squeezed tightly.

The rain continued to fall, but we just sat there quietly together. Cold, wet, and miserable, but together.

After sitting in the rain for far too long, Emma decided to go home to dry off. We said a soggy good-bye with a big hug and a kiss at the park gates, then went our separate ways. I felt so awful leaving her—watching her walk away from me on her own, knowing what she was going through—but I also felt that I needed some time on my own to digest everything she'd said and collect my thoughts. I wasn't being any use to her gobsmacked and teary, unable to utter a single sensible word.

And so I went home, lay down on my bed, and stared at the four walls of my bedroom, going over and over in my mind what Emma had told me. I heard Mr. Davies come indoors from smoking his pipe in the garden as usual, pop it back in the drawer, and settle down for the night in front of the telly. Life was going on as normal.

I couldn't understand how Emma could possibly be HIV positive. It didn't make sense. How could my cousin have HIV? One day she was walking around perfectly fine and the next she was telling me that she had got some hideous life-threatening disease. It just didn't seem real. You only ever hear stories like this on GMTV. The family sits on the sofa to tell the nation their sad story and everyone shakes their heads in dismay saying things like "Tragic" and "So young" and "She had her whole life ahead of her." But this wasn't some break-fast TV scenario, this was actually happening to my cousin Emma. I couldn't get my head around it.

I felt really confused. I didn't know anything about HIV or AIDS, and I had so many questions that I didn't know where to start. All I knew about HIV was stuff I'd heard at school from friends or in our stupid sex education class when Mr. Allan, our biology teacher, put on a video and then hid at the back of the class so that we couldn't see how embarrassed he got. He wouldn't take questions at the end, so any queries we had went unanswered and we were all left guessing. I can remember them talking about sexually transmitted diseases in the video, and HIV was one of the diseases you could catch if you didn't have safe sex.

I thought it was only gay men who could get HIV, though. That's what everyone said after the class, anyway. That's why Colin in our year, who is really girlie and always gets teased for being gay, was thrown in the pond by a bunch of lads who'd shouted that he'd got AIDS and wasn't welcome in our school.

I decided to go downtown to see how Em was first thing the next morning. I was sure she'd think I'd blurted everything out to my parents or that I'd never talk to her again. I just needed to see her and reassure her that I was there for her and that I always would be. I was worried that I was going to start acting differently around her or something. I just wanted things to be normal.

THREE

THE SMELL OF THE TRADITIONAL SUNDAY FRIED breakfast—sausages, bacon, black pudding, eggs, beans: the whole heart-stopping lot—wafted upstairs and woke me up. I shoved on the clothes that I'd left at the side of my bed the night before and wandered downstairs to get myself a cup of tea and make the usual pleasantries before I could successfully leave to see Emma without too many questions being asked. On the way down I noticed another new little pearl of wisdom above the phone at the bottom of the stairs. Written in neat calligraphy behind a rose-pink frame, it said SMILE AND THE WORLD SMILES WITH YOU.

Mum acquired a taste for these New Age proverbs after a ladies' night at a friend's house a few months ago. Her friend Margaret had held an aromatherapy party in her living room and had presented all of her guests with a fridge magnet. Each one said something like: THERE HAVE BEEN TIMES WHEN YOU HAVE HAD ENOUGH CARES OF YOUR OWN AND YET YOU CARED. "It's all the rage," Mum had said. She doesn't usually go out anywhere, but the promise of coming home with a basket of scented floating candles and some knickknacks for the bathroom had been too much to resist. Ever since, anything that had one of those life-enhancing, self-confidence-boosting messages would be snapped up and placed strategically about the house. As a result, there's a lace toilet-roll cover in the bathroom with the embroidered message CHERISH YESTERDAY, DREAM TOMORROW, LIVE TODAY, and a framed tapestry— ACTION MAY NOT ALWAYS BE HAPPINESS, BUT THERE IS NO HAPPINESS WITHOUT ACTION—hanging on the kitchen wall. I'm not sure whether Mum takes much notice of the actual messages; as long as they match the curtains or the wallpaper, up they go.

"Morning, Leyla. Fancy a fry-up?" Mum asked, balancing a piece of crispy bacon on a spatula in front of my face.

"Mum, how many times have I got to tell you? I'm vegetarian."

"You don't know what you're missing. These pigs were bred to be eaten. They don't know any different."

"Mum, you're making my head hurt. Pass me the orange juice."

"Please."

"Pleeese."

Dad was sat at the kitchen table reading the *Mail on Sunday,* muttering to himself, shaking his head from side to side, a look of utter dismay on his face.

"What's with the long face, Dad? Another famine in Sudan? Another fatal plane crash?" I said sarcastically.

"No, Man City has lost again," he tutted.

Swigging down the last of my orange juice, desperate to get to Emma's, I grabbed my coat, which was still damp from the day before, and ran out of the back door, shouting, "I'm going out. Won't be long."

I got to the chemist, with its window display of cheap perfume, and remembered the time Emma worked there on Saturdays for the formidable Mrs. Granger. Emma was always in all sorts of trouble. One day a hulky, fifteen-stone builder wearing overalls and a hard hat, covered from head to toe in cement dust, came into the shop and asked Emma if they sold face masks. She led him to the end of the shop and talked him through all the different types of exfoliating, moisturizing, cleansing face masks they had on offer. When Emma asked him if he had combination, dry, or greasy skin, he asked her if she was taking the piss, then marched up to the main desk to complain to Mrs. Granger.

Emma, totally amused by all the fuss, was given a lecture on her sarcastic and smarmy attitude and told to shape up or ship out. Still none the wiser as to what she had done wrong, Emma listened to Mrs. Granger explain that the builder had wanted a mask to cover his mouth to stop all the dust from the construction site getting in. Emma's snort of laughter infuriated Mrs. Granger even more, and Emma was given her marching orders. It was the final straw, according to Mrs. Granger; Emma could apparently not take her job seriously and would have to go.

I laughed to myself remembering the story and ran up the stairs to the flat, eager to see Emma. Aunty Jean opened the door with a cigarette in her mouth, wearing a peach satin dressing gown that had gone bobbly from too much wear and too many washes. She looked terrible, absolutely shattered. Her hair looked as though it hadn't been washed for quite a few days. Our eyes met. There was a blankness in hers. Their usual sparkle had disappeared. She knew instantly that I knew. We didn't say anything for a moment and then, putting on a false smile, she waved me inside.

"You're an early bird. Do you want some breakfast, darling? How's your mum? Cleaning the house, I bet. She doesn't let a speck of dust settle for two seconds in that house. I don't know where she gets it from, 'cos your granny wasn't like that, I can tell you. We lived in a pigsty growing up, we did. Fancy some orange juice?"

"I'm all right, thanks. Where's Em?" I said quickly, keen to make a sharp exit.

Aunty Jean had drifted off and was staring out of the kitchen window. Her face looked drawn and her mouth tight and pursed. I could see the lines around her lips and the dark shadows around her eyes. She's usually the life and soul of the party, just like Emma. It was weird to see her so quiet and distant. Aunty Jean is always the one to fill the silences, crack the jokes, make you smile when you're down. She's the complete opposite of my mum. Mum is so sensible. She abides by so many unwritten rules as to how she thinks "one" should behave.

All of Emma's friends love Aunty Jean, because she's so open and friendly and you can talk to her about anything. She gives us a glass of wine on the weekend and lets us stay up late to watch whatever films on TV we like. I've always wished Mum were more like her. Emma talks to her mum about sex and boyfriends and everything. My mum turns the telly off if so much as a naked buttock comes on the screen. That's probably why Emma was able to tell Aunty Jean about the HIV, though I don't think anything could have prepared her for Emma's news. It was so strange to see her all quiet and withdrawn. It made me feel really uncomfortable, and I just wanted to get out of there.

"Aunty Jean, where's Em?" I said, a little louder this time.

"Oh sorry, love, I was miles away. She's in the bath. She's been in there for ages, though. She'll be like a prune by now. Go and bang on the door and get her out of there, will you?"

As I walked down the narrow hallway, I could feel myself shaking. Why hadn't I hugged Aunty Jean and told her how sorry I was, shared my confusion and fears and grief with her? I'd just clammed up the minute I saw her. I could feel my throat tighten and the palms of my hands begin to sweat. I've known her all my life; she's like my second mum. Why did I suddenly feel so awkward and shy around her? It's times like these that you really need the people close to you, but I'd shut myself off from her.

What was I going to be like with Emma? I just wanted to run away and pretend none of this was happening. I was faltering outside the bathroom door when Emma burst out and banged straight into me.

"Where did *you* come from? You scared the living daylights out of me. What are you doing here so early anyway?"

I followed her into her bright orange bedroom. It felt like stepping into the center of the sun with the early morning light shining through the orange curtains, which matched the orange bedspread, orange walls, and orange rug.

"I was worried about you. I haven't slept a wink." I was looking down at my hands, too scared to make eye contact in case I started crying or she saw the fear in my eyes.

"Oh Leyla, don't worry. I'm fine. Look at me—I'm

fighting fit." She rolled up her dressing gown sleeves and flexed her muscles in a mock-muscleman pose.

She looked awful. Not ill or anything, just white and washed out, with these terrible big bags under her eyes. In fact, her eyes looked dead, the same as Aunty Jean's. I was sure she was making light of things because she felt uncomfortable talking to me about it and was worried about what I was thinking. I wanted to break down the barriers that I knew we were both building between us, but I didn't know how.

"Well, I just wanted you to know that I won't ever disown you or abandon you. I just want you to be okay. It's so awful. I . . . I . . ."

I slumped down on her bed and started crying. I hadn't meant to at all. Emma put her arm around me and started comforting me, which seemed completely ridiculous and wrong.

"I'm the one who's supposed to be comforting you," I sobbed.

FOUR

EMMA DECIDED THAT WE BOTH NEEDED TO GO OUT
for some fresh air, and so we headed down to the bit of the
park where kids hang out in the games arcade and families
hire splash cats for a jolly day out on the lake.

We got two bottles of Coke from the kiosk and sat on a
bench to drink them. Looking down at her hands in her lap,
twisting a soggy tissue round and round her little finger,
Emma proceeded to tell me the sequence of events that had
led to her finding out she was HIV positive. I wasn't aware of
anything or anyone else around us.

"Do you remember when I went on that stupid school trip
to Wales in January and we stayed in that youth hostel in the
mountains for a week?"

"Oh yeah, and it rained every day and you phoned home
practically every night, bored out of your brain."

"Yep, that's the one. On our last night the youth hostel organized a disco for us and some other schools that were staying there. It was awful. Cheesy dance anthems playing all night, bad fashion everywhere I looked, and loads of girls on one side of the room giggling and twittering away in cliques while glancing over to the other side of the room where the boys were congregated, gagging for some action. You could have sliced the sexual tension with a blunt knife.

"Well, anyway, I was bored stupid. Me and Jo were sat talking in the corner when these two lads from a school in Birmingham came up to us and asked if we wanted to go outside with them for a drink, as they had a couple of bottles of wine stashed away. Jo was reluctant at first, but I managed to persuade her and off we went. Before we knew it we were plastered, laughing our heads off, having sunk a big bottle of red wine between us. I should have seen what was coming; it was so obvious. One of the guys started kissing my neck while we were sat on a fence at the edge of the woods behind the youth hostel. It felt quite nice, and we ended up snogging.

"Well, you can guess what happened next. We both got extremely carried away and led each other off to where it was dark and secluded. I suppose I felt I deserved a bit of fun after serving a whole week in purgatory, stuck in the middle of nowhere. It was funny, because he was wearing these awful Y-fronts that I just couldn't stop laughing at when he took his trousers off. And then . . . you know, we had sex."

"But you didn't use anything."

"No. I was so swept away by the moment that I didn't want it to be ruined by having to stop and hunt around for some condoms. I knew exactly what I was doing. I remember telling myself that it would be okay not to use a condom just this once and promised myself that I'd never do it again. I did quite enjoy myself with him. I mean, he was gorgeous, but it was just five minutes' worth of sex in a drunken tangle that wouldn't even be memorable if it weren't for this . . . this mess. Can you believe it? All I wanted was a bit of fun, and I got a life sentence. Those five minutes in the woods with some sad Brummie bloke have shaped the rest of my life. What a mess. What an unbelievable mess."

She broke down, curled her head between her knees, and sobbed. I really didn't know what to say; I'd never felt so small and helpless in my life. All I could do was sit there and hold her and make sure she knew I was there with her. Resting her head on my lap, combing my fingers through her hair, I sat and cried with her. It felt as though I'd done little else but cry for the past twenty-four hours, and I was beginning to feel totally drained.

It seemed like hours had passed when Emma eventually lifted her head, wiped her face with her sleeve, and slowly drew herself to her feet.

"Come on, Leyla, let's just go for a walk. I'm sick of sitting around crying all the time. I've done nothing else for months."

We got up and walked, not thinking about where we were going. I had so many questions I wanted to ask Emma, but I was worried that I would upset her or that she just wanted to talk about normal stuff and forget about everything else. But she carried on talking about how awful it had been when she found out her results, so I thought it would be okay to ask her some things.

"What made you go for an HIV test in the first place, though, Em? I mean, I know loads of girls at school who brag about having had sex without a condom, and I'm sure it's never crossed their minds to go and get tested."

"It's quite a long story really."

"Listen, if you don't want to talk about it now, just say. Just tell me to shut up if you want."

"No, it's okay, I don't mind. It's such a relief to talk about it openly with someone. It's difficult talking to my mum all the time. She gets so upset; it's hard to handle. I feel as though I'm driving a dagger through her heart every time I mention it. She only has to look in my eyes and she bursts into tears. I feel so guilty for putting her through all of this. If I hadn't been so stupid I wouldn't be hurting her the way I am."

"Oh, Em, don't blame yourself. So many girls have unprotected sex all the time and just cross their fingers hoping that they'll be all right, that they won't get pregnant or catch some disease. You never think you'll be the unlucky one, do you? We're all convinced that it may happen to someone else but never to yours truly. Your mum isn't blaming you. Anyway, that boy has got a lot to answer for."

"I can't even think about him yet. I don't know where to begin. I'm blocking all of that out. I can't think about him."

"So, what made you go for the test then?"

"You know that girl Susie I've told you about who was in my school? She lives in the big house on the corner of your estate and everyone in the world fancies her?"

"Yeah, I know the one."

"Well, she hates running because she's got quite big boobs and she says they hurt when she runs, and I love any excuse not to do cross-country, so we always end up being running, or should I say 'strolling' partners so that we can skive off and take all the shortcuts. We used to walk most of the way and end up chatting quite a lot. Anyway, one day we were talking about boys and sex and everything, and she mentioned that she had got what she thought was really bad thrush and didn't know what to do about it. I told her that I'd been to a well-woman clinic with my mum because she had to get a smear test done and while I was waiting for her to have the test I picked up some leaflets in the waiting room, which were all about things like thrush, chlamydia, cystitis, and all those women's problems. I said that I'd go down there with her to keep her company if she wanted me to.

"Anyway, after talking for ages about boys and who we fancied it turns out she'd had sex with this guy from the boys' school and hadn't used anything and had started worrying about all sorts of things like HIV and everything, as this guy had a huge reputation for sleeping around a lot and people had been teasing her—saying that she'd probably caught something nasty off him. That's when I started getting really paranoid about what had happened in Wales. I told her about the boy at the youth hostel and we eventually made a pact to go to the clinic together and both get HIV tests and sort out her thrush at the same time.

"When I got home I read through the leaflets I'd picked up and they said you could get confidential HIV tests done at a GUM clinic—genitourinary medicine, I think it stands for—where you didn't even have to give your real name if you didn't want to. I decided that it would be better to go there since they'd seen me at the well-woman clinic with my mum. I didn't want anyone to recognize me."

"I'd never have enough guts to go and get an HIV test. I'd be too embarrassed."

"We didn't take it that seriously. We just thought we'd go

and get a full MOT to put our minds at rest and we'd never have unprotected sex again and everything would be hunky-dory." Emma took a deep breath and let out a long exasperated sigh. The tears were welling up in her eyes. I had to bite the inside of my cheek to stop myself from crying again. I knew I had to be strong for her. She had enough on her plate without me blubbing on her shoulder twice in one day.

"The GUM clinic is in the Manchester Royal Infirmary, so we got on the tram and went into Manchester after school one day," Emma continued. "We each saw a woman doctor privately. Mine took me into this room and explained how the test would be done and how the result would be given. She said that it would be completely confidential and that not even my GP would know about it. I was glad about that, because I was worried my mum might hear about it if I called the hospital. You know what they're like in that place. People go there just for the gossip, not because they're ill."

"But I saw you coming out of the doctor's last week, remember, when your mum said you had flu."

"Well, she knew by then, and it turns out that there's a doctor at the surgery who has done a load of research into HIV treatments, so I made an appointment with him just to see what he was like."

"But before she knew anything, weren't you worried that your mum would open your mail or take a message from the clinic and ask you what it was all about?"

"No. The woman told me that they never give out results over the phone or by letter; I'd have to go back to the clinic in person a week later to collect the results.

"She asked me all these questions about why I thought I might have HIV, why I wanted the test in the first place, and asked me to describe my sexual and drug-taking history. They basically wanted to find out if I'd really thought through having a test. By my talking about my sexual history they could see whether I was really at risk of having HIV or not. They want you to take the test seriously; I can see why now. And then, after we'd talked for a while about everything, she asked me if I still wanted the test."

"I would have run away, I know I would have. I just wouldn't have had the guts to go through with it."

"Well, by that point, after talking about it and realizing how stupid I'd been, I just wanted to have the checkup. I never thought the result would be positive, so I thought that if I had the test done I could put it behind me and just get on with my life. As I'd made all the effort to go to the clinic in the first place, I thought that I might as well, seeing as I was there.

"The woman said that when someone is infected with HIV it can take as long as three months to show up on an HIV test. Well, I went on the school trip to Wales in January, and by the time I went to the clinic it was the end of the summer term in June—I'd just had my last exam—so it was well over three months. But before she actually took the blood test she said that she thought we ought to discuss what the result might be and how I would cope, whatever the result. She asked me if I had close friends and family I could talk to and if there was anyone I could bring back to the clinic with me for support when I had to collect the results and whether I was prepared for whatever the results might be. God, there were so many questions. I mean, I appreciate it now—they were so thorough and so supportive—but at the time I can remember checking my watch and wishing they'd hurry up or I'd miss *Hollyoaks*.

"When the test was over I met Susie in the waiting room and we got the tram home together before saying good-bye, then I rushed off to watch TV."

"So you had to go back a week later to get the results. Did you go with Susie?"

"No, I saw her in school a few days later and she told me that she wasn't going to bother going back for her results. They'd given her some cream and pessaries for her thrush and it seemed to be clearing up and that was all she was bothered about. I told her that I probably wasn't going to go back either and had just gone along for the experience and to keep her company."

"How come you went back? Did you go on your own?"

"I couldn't stop thinking about the results, I suppose. I'd gone through all the hassle of having the test done, so I thought I might as well go and get confirmation that I was all clear. I never thought in a million years that the results would be positive, and I wasn't prepared for it, no matter how much I'd managed to convince the doctor at the clinic that I was. I also thought that I could just stock up on a load of free condoms while I was there, because I had vowed to myself never to have unprotected sex again.

"So, I went back a week later on my own. I didn't tell Susie I was going and I didn't want to get anybody else involved, as I thought I could keep the whole thing my little secret. I got to the clinic and the same doctor took me into a private room and told me that she had some very difficult news to tell me. And she broke it to me there and then that the results were positive. And, well, I've told you the rest. I asked for my mum to come to the clinic, and that was it."

We both gazed off into the distance, taking everything in.

I was amazed Emma still had enough energy to tell me the whole story after everything she'd been through.

"My throat's all dry from all this talking. I'm fed up with talking now, Leyla. Shall we do something else instead?" Emma asked, breaking the silence.

It took me a while to click into action, I was so stunned by it all. I felt numb, but my brain was racing, trying to make sense of what she'd said. Sensing, though, that Emma needed to take her mind off things, I snapped out of it and suggested we do something I hadn't done in a long while.

"Let's get a splash cat. Come on, I haven't been on one since I was little," I urged. "A swan came up to the side where I was sat and pecked my bum so hard I couldn't sit down for a week afterward."

"Great. Sounds like fun," Emma said, rolling her eyes and challenging me to a race back to the kiosk.

FIVE

IT HAD BEEN ALMOST A MONTH SINCE EMMA TOLD me that she was HIV positive. I still hadn't stopped thinking about her every second of the day, worrying about her so much I couldn't sleep properly. My best mate Sarah had been trying to wheedle out of me why I'd been so tired and distracted, and in an effort to cheer me up she'd bought me a ticket to see Asian Dub Foundation at the Academy, chaperoned by her older brother Jamie.

It was Friday night and I had been given strict instructions to be wearing my party hat—to be ready for a big one. But walking down to Sarah's through my estate I couldn't help but think of the leaflets I had read at school that day in the nurse's office. I'd found them tucked behind the leaflets on healthy eating and on smoking. There was a whole bundle of fact sheets on HIV and AIDS that you'd never have known were there unless you were looking. I read that ten thousand teenagers in Britain are living with or are affected by HIV.

I couldn't believe what I was reading. Where were they all? How come we didn't hear about it on the news or read about it in the newspapers? Why this veil of secrecy? Why hadn't we ever heard anyone talk about teenagers with HIV in school? We were always being asked to raise money for children with leukemia or severe disabilities and were taught to act compassionately and generously toward those less fortunate than ourselves. So why didn't we hear about all the kids living with HIV and AIDS?

I thought of Emma and Aunty Jean not being able to talk to friends or family about Emma's illness and having to battle against it all on their own. I'd begun to learn how much prejudice there was around HIV. People don't want to talk about it. They're scared they might catch it just from breathing the same air as someone who is HIV positive. Nobody realizes that there are people like Emma out there who have just had a bit of bad luck from one careless mistake. She didn't mean any harm. Thinking about all this made me so angry I didn't realize how fast I was walking, and before I knew it I was at Sarah's.

"Hello, Leyla. Come on in, dear. It's cold out there tonight. It gets so dark so early now, doesn't it? It's hard to get used to it after the long summer days—well, if you can call it summer. They don't call Manchester the rainy city for nothing, that's for sure." Mrs. Powell ushered me in to number twenty-four, fussing over me, hanging up my coat properly. She is dead religious and has got crucifixes and pictures of Jesus and the Virgin Mary all over the walls in the hallway. They freak me out. Mary's eyes seem to follow you wherever you go in the house.

Mrs. Powell despairs of Sarah and is always desperately trying to get her to lead a good Catholic way of life. But Sarah's having none of it. The only icon she can be bothered to worship is Madonna. Once she cut out hundreds of pictures of Madonna's head from different magazines and stuck them all over her mum's pictures of Jesus so that it was the singer who was sacrificed on the cross to save us from evil. Her mum stopped Sarah's allowance for months for that blasphemy and literally dragged her to church every Sunday for weeks on end.

As I stood in the hall watching Mrs. Powell negotiate my coat onto a hanger, I wondered what she'd have to say about Emma. She always asked after Em because she'd wanted Sarah to go to the same convent as Emma, but Sarah refused, not wanting to be separated from me. Aunty Jean had only sent Em there because she was keen for her to get good grades and thought the convent would be the best place for her.

I knew Mrs. Powell would be really upset about Em being ill, because she's such a lovely, kind woman who wouldn't wish anybody any harm. But I'm sure she'd freak to think that Em was having sex before marriage in the first place. And she wouldn't be thinking about whether Emma could have prevented herself from catching anything by having safe sex, because strict Catholics don't agree with contraception anyway. I wonder if she'd think the disease was a punishment for having sex before marriage, full stop. But then what would she think about babies who are born with HIV after contracting it from their mothers or people who get it from blood transfusions? Were those people innocent victims? Was there some sort of hierarchy, with "sinners," who don't deserve real compassion at the bottom, and "innocents" at the top? It was all too confusing, too complicated.

"She's getting ready in her room," Sarah's mum said, pointing up the stairs. "I haven't heard a peep out of her for at least an hour. I don't know what she's getting up to."

I ran up the stairs like I had done since I was eight years old and Sarah had become my best friend at primary school. Our friendship started when she helped me out of a particularly sticky situation that involved me being on the front line of the animal liberation movement for the first time as I set the school hamster free. She took the flak, and I've been in her debt ever since.

Sarah's always been bold and up front. She won't take any shit from anyone, having learnt to stand up for herself when she was little and being teased to death all the time because of her fiery red hair. When we went up to the high school she decided to dye it black, and I haven't seen her natural color since. At the moment it's black with bleached blond streaks that are pink on the tips. She looks incredible. She reckons she's fat and out of proportion, but she's just your classic pear shape: quite small with broad hips and petite on top. She's still dead paranoid and insecure about her looks, though, and tries to detract attention from her body by being smart-arsed and cheeky all the time. She's also as neurotic as hell. For instance, she won't have a bath unless it's on the hour. She'll phone me up and have nothing to say because she's just passing a little bit of time until the clock strikes the hour so she can go and have a bath. I've told her she needs to get some help.

I barged straight into her room without knocking, as usual, only this time I got something I hadn't bargained for: Sarah was lying stark naked on her bed, wrapped from head to toe in cling film.

"I wish you'd knock," she said from her horizontal position.

The shock of finding my best friend wrapped like an Egyptian mummy in transparent plastic floored me.

"What are you doing? What the hell are you doing?" I managed to croak between peals of laughter.

"Don't just stand there gawping, help me get this stuff off. There are some scissors on the dressing table." I began snipping away at the cling film as she explained how she'd got herself in such a ridiculous state. "I was reading my mum's *Woman's Own* last night in the toilet and saw this article about alternative ways of getting rid of a few extra pounds, and one of them was to wrap yourself up in cling film and sweat some weight off. Can't say it's had much effect, though. My skin feels gross. I just wanted to be able to squeeze into my denim skirt for tonight."

As soon as she was free of her plastic casing she got into her dressing gown and headed for the bathroom. "Come and talk to me while I'm in the shower."

The magazine in question was open on her bedside table, so I had a quick read. "You're absolutely bonkers. You don't need to lose weight, for a start, and if you'd read the article properly you'd have noticed that it said you should only do it in controlled conditions with an expert beautician or someone like that on hand. You're barking mad, you are." I sat on the toilet while Sarah had her shower, and in the hot, steamy atmosphere of the bathroom let my mind drift off again.

"Sarah," I suddenly said, "have you ever thought about what it must be like to be really, really ill or know that someone really close to you, like your mum or dad, was dying?"

"Oh my God, bundle of laughs *you* are tonight," Sarah shouted incredulously from the shower cubicle. "Don't be so morbid. What's got into you lately? It's Friday night and we're going to the gig of the century. What are you like?" Sarah wiped the steam from the shower door and stared at me through the glass with a stern warning in her eyes that told me to cheer up and get in the mood.

I was really looking forward to the gig, and I knew that moping around wasn't going to help Emma in any way, but I just couldn't seem to drag myself out of it. I wanted to blurt everything out to Sarah. It was the first time I'd ever hidden anything from her; we told each other everything usually. But I knew I had to be careful what I said to her because although she's my best friend and I'd trust her with my life, I'd vowed to Emma not to tell another soul. I knew the consequences could be devastating. People are so ignorant about HIV that if gossip spread I was sure Emma would be forced out of school by small-minded bullies. But I didn't see any harm in talking to Sarah about the issue in general.

"I know, I know. I am looking forward to tonight. I'm not depressed or anything, I was just wondering what it must feel like to have a really serious illness like cancer or HIV or something like that and to know that you were dying. You heard what Mr. Strong was saying in assembly the other day about how much we'd raised for all those kids with leukemia. It must be so weird being our age and wanting to plan for the future but not actually knowing whether you're going to be alive that long. Don't you ever feel completely helpless? Like there are so many problems in this world and so many people suffering and you can't do a thing about it?"

"Well, I don't lose too much sleep over it, to be honest, Leyla. I tend to concentrate more on how I'm going to get some beautiful rich guy to sweep me off my feet one day."

I could tell Sarah was getting frustrated with me, and so I

decided to try to put things out of my mind for the night and concentrate on having a good time.

Sarah's older brother Jamie shouted up the stairs to tell us he was leaving in ten minutes. He was going to the gig with his best mate Lee and was driving us all there in his VW camper. As we piled into the van, I could see Sarah's mother at the lounge window mouthing to Jamie to drive carefully. Sarah and I flopped down on the mattress in the back and Jamie cranked up the stereo, then sped up as soon as we were out of his mum's sight.

The excitement of being in the back of the van with my best mate, music blaring and the fresh night air blowing in through the windows, gave me a real buzz and got me back on track. I thought how I could live quite happily in a van like this and just travel round the world doing as I pleased, parking up wherever took my fancy. I'd never have to listen to Sadie's mundane routines or my mum's nagging again. I'd be as free as a bird.

I looked over at Sarah, who was putting the finishing touches on her makeup in a hand mirror, and thought how good it felt to be heading out on the town for a mad night out. Sarah looked fantastic in her knee-length denim skirt, black leather boots, and black leather bomber jacket. And I was wearing my new Indian print top that showed my midriff so you could see my belly-button ring. We looked great, and I suddenly felt invincible. There we were singing at the tops of our voices, speeding into Manchester, ready for some big fun. I felt alive and special. Mum and Sadie wouldn't have a clue what it was like to feel this untouchable, like I could do anything, be anyone, go anywhere.

As we arrived in the center of Manchester, I could feel the

buzz from down the road even before we reached the venue. This was my favorite kind of night out. I loved seeing live bands, feeling the energy of the music and the crowd, and going bonkers down at the front, emerging sweaty and exhausted after having risked my life just to be able to say that I'd been there, by the stage, and the lead singer had winked at me. Of course, after every gig I've ever been to I've gone home saying that the lead singer waved, winked, blew me a kiss, or whispered something in my ear.

Inside the Academy, despite strict instructions from Sarah's mum not to let us out of their sight, Jamie and Lee decided to ditch their "younger and geekier hangers-on." They left us the minute we walked in the doors and told us to meet them by the T-shirt stall when it was all over. Sarah was bouncing up and down on the spot with excitement, her eyes darting everywhere, chewing furiously on her gum, soaking up the atmosphere and intensity of the gig that was about to begin.

"Go and get us a couple of drinks, will you, Leyla?"

"I probably won't get served but I'll try. What do you fancy?"

"Champagne, tequila, Jack Daniel's—whatever you can get your underage mittens on."

"Okay, here goes."

Pushing my way up to the packed bar, trying to put on some more lippy without smudging it all over my face as I went, I spotted a group of people from sixth form. I vaguely knew one of them, Darren; he used to be in the school orchestra with me. But I wasn't sure if he'd recognize me, so I tried not to make eye contact. The next thing I knew I was jostled around so much in the crowd at the bar that I was rubbing elbows with him.

A flicker of recognition passed over his face. "All right? You're from Bishops High, aren't you?"

"Yeah, you used to be in the orchestra, didn't you?" I said shyly.

"Oh yeah, that's it. You play the drums. You were always bashing away making some impressive sounds while I screeched the whole orchestra to a halt on that bloody violin of mine. Who are you with?"

"My friend Sarah and her brother Jamie—Jamie Powell. He was in the year above you. He finished his A Levels this summer."

"Oh yeah, I know Jamie. He drives around in that clapped-out VW, doesn't he?"

"Yeah, we've just come down in it. It's cool actually, I love it. It's got a fridge, a bed, and a sink in it. You'd never need to go home if you didn't want to."

My heart was going like the clappers. Darren was gorgeous. He had short dark hair that was slightly longer on top and waxed into a mini Mohican down the middle of his head. He was wearing a white T-shirt with capped sleeves that showed off a little swallow tattoo on his upper right arm. He had really long dark eyelashes and green eyes that sent me drifting off into la-la land when I looked into them—until I was jolted back to reality by the bar attendant asking for my order.

"Two vodka and oranges please," I said as confidently as possible.

She reached for the glasses then looked at me again and hesitated. "You're not eighteen, are you?"

Darren was still stood right next to me. I wanted the ground to open up and swallow me. "Yes, I am," I muttered weakly.

"Show us your ID then."

"Umm, I've left it at home. I'm never usually asked. It was my eighteenth in August."

"Sorry. No ID, no booze. Next please." She moved on to the next person.

I could feel my cheeks burning up and I thought I'd die of embarrassment. I wanted to crawl back to Sarah and pretend that nothing had happened, but Darren grabbed my arm just as I was turning away from the bar and told me to wait over by the pillar for him. Next thing, he was tapping me on the shoulder gesturing me to take a couple of drinks out of his hands.

"There you go—two vodka and oranges. I'm not sure I approve of underage drinking, but what the hell, it'll put hairs on your chest." He winked at me, raised his glass in a toast— "Here's to a top night"—and walked off toward his mates before I'd even had a chance to say thank you.

The concert was mind-blowing. Sarah and I were so close to the band we could practically see the lead singer's nasal hairs. Sarah kept grabbing his trouser leg to try to get his attention. I was hoping that Darren would be down the front as well and kept looking out for him, but didn't see him at all. He was probably being cool at the back and would turn his nose up if he saw me getting so sweaty and disheveled.

After it was all over, while we were waiting for Jamie and Lee to appear at the T-shirt stall, I thought about the gig and how fantastic it must be to be in a successful band: doing exactly what you always wanted to do with your life every day, playing live in front of an adoring audience in a different city every night. It must be so exciting. The energy and reckless-ness of the gig made me come out in goose pimples just thinking about it. I so desperately want to be up on stage playing my drums.

The thought that I might end up working in a building society like my sister when I leave school makes me feel physically ill. All I want to do is play my drums. I don't want to waste any time doing the sensible thing with my life: getting a career, planning for my future with kids and a family to look after, getting a pension, building a nest egg. Knowing what's happened to Emma has made me realize that anything can happen and you might as well live life to the full while you've got the chance to.

I'm going to grab life by the balls. The blokes who work in the music shop in Bury tease me all the time for playing the drums. They say I should leave drumming to the boys. When I talk about being in a band and going on tour they laugh their heads off, saying that I wouldn't have the stamina to last a full-length gig because I'm a girl and not tough enough. They're so full of shit. I'll show them. As long as you've got passion and faith and are willing to work hard, you can do anything you want in this life, I reckon.

SIX

AT SCHOOL, ON THE MONDAY AFTER THE GIG, I HEADED straight to Sarah and my secret hiding place during first break and met Sarah there. Underneath the stage in the main hall there's a basement area where they store old costumes from shows the school has put on, and all sorts of props and old desks and shelving units. You go down some steps at the side of the stage and through a tiny little door that opens up into this huge storage area full of old junk that no one is particularly bothered about. The door is never locked, so we use it as our special place where we can get away from everyone and talk without being disturbed. Sarah's always messing around with whatever she can find down there, and when I walked in she was sat reading a magazine and wearing a nun's habit left over from a production of *The Sound of Music*. Impersonating her mum at church on a Sunday, she blessed me as I made myself comfortable on a bag of clothes and asked me to repent all of my sins.

"We'd be here all day," I said, chuckling.

We were in the middle of dissecting Friday night's gig, discussing which song we'd liked the best, when we heard someone outside trying the door handle and attempting to push their way in. We both jumped to our feet, hearts pounding, grabbed our bags, and tried to scramble together an excuse as to why we were in there.

We were sure it was a teacher who was about to discover us, but as the door opened and I prepared to launch into a spiel about how we needed to be in there as it was a quiet space to finish off some homework, Darren's gorgeous face appeared round the door.

"What the hell are you wearing?" he said, pointing at Sarah.

We dropped our bags and let out huge sighs of relief. Sarah slumped back down to the floor and pulled off the nun's habit. I grabbed Darren by his school tie and pulled him in so that he wasn't half in, half out and in view of anybody passing by.

"What are you doing here? Have you been following us?" I was surprised at how fast my heart was beating and how glad I was to see him. I hadn't really thought about him that much over the weekend, but seeing him again made me realize how much I actually fancied him.

"I saw you coming out of the biology lab before break and spotted you heading in this direction. I was curious to see where you were going when I saw you come into the main hall. Do you always come here?"

"Yeah, we like to come here to be on our own. We don't usually have many guests, actually, and when we do they're formally invited." I was being cocky and self-assured, worried that he might be able to see right through me and spot the fact that my heart was slowly turning into a gooey mess in his presence. Pathetic, I know.

"Yeah, if we'd known you were coming we'd have baked a cake," Sarah said frostily.

"Ouch! I thought Mother Teresa was supposed to show kindness and generosity at all times toward her fellow human beings. I did get you those drinks on Friday night, remember? Surely I deserve a better reception than this."

"Okay, okay, sit down. You've got to promise not to tell anyone that we come here, though, or we'll have nowhere to get away from the idiots in our year." I didn't want him to think that we were totally unwelcoming.

"Don't worry, your Wendy house secret is safe with me."

"Oi, you, it's not a Wendy house, and if you're going to disrespect our space you can leave," Sarah barked.

"Easy! Easy! Okay, I'm sorry. The reason I followed you in here in the first place was to tell you that I'm DJing for a friend's party at a new bar in Bury on Saturday night and I wondered whether you two wanted to come along."

He handed us a couple of flyers and told us that he hoped to see us there. As he walked out the door he turned round and, tapping his forefinger to the side of his nose, said, "Mum's the word."

As soon as I thought he was out of earshot, I let out a huge groan. "He is *so* fit."

"He's a bit of a dick, I reckon."

"God, he's gorgeous." I was deaf to Sarah's comments.

There was just something about Darren that sent sparks flying inside my head. I barely knew him, but just being around him made my stomach flip over. "We've got to go to that party on Saturday night. It's not often we get invited to things by that older crowd. And besides, I want to know why Darren was so interested in finding out where I was going when he saw me today."

"You fancy the pants off him, don't you? He's too smug, Leyla. He doesn't need you to fancy him—he fancies himself enough already. The way he came swanning in here thinking that we'd be so impressed that he's DJing on Saturday. Why does he think we'd be so interested in going to some crappy party with him anyway?"

"Oh, and have you got anything better to do? We're going and that's final."

Sarah was saved by the bell from having to commit herself. Still, I knew there would be no stopping her. She's never missed the opportunity of a party. Round here, the council's idea of keeping teenagers entertained is a piddly dry ski slope on the side of an old slag heap, so you never miss a party when you're invited.

"Come on, we'd better go, it's sports next. Your favorite!" Sarah said, springing to her feet and dusting herself off.

I loathe sport. Throwing a ball around a pitch or court seems the most pointless exercise in the world to me, especially during winter when it's cold enough to freeze your nipples off. It's such a waste of time. It was the beginning of November, subzero temperatures outside, and we had to stand in a court in skimpy netball skirts while Mrs. Rose, the PE teacher, shouted abuse from the sidelines, all wrapped up warm in her cozy, powder blue tracksuit that matched the eye shadow reaching all the way up to her perfectly plucked eyebrows, giving her a look of constant surprise.

Only moving when I was in danger of being knocked unconscious by a spinning netball hurtling toward my head, I was even more distracted than usual by thoughts of the delectable Darren. Was he really interested in me? Had he made a point of following me from biology because he actually liked me or was he just being naturally friendly? Or did he like Sarah?

I was so wrapped up in these thoughts that it took me a while to realize the game had in fact come to a halt—Mrs. Rose had been called over to the hockey pitch because of an injury. Instead of carrying on the game, Claire Higgins, the "It" girl of our year, and her cronies were beginning to close in on Teresa Glass and tease her about her brown front teeth and rotting gums.

Taking a few slow steps backward to the fence, I edged away from the situation, reluctant to get involved. Claire Higgins slinked about the court, dressed head to toe in designer Nike gear. She's got long brown permed hair that she scrunch-dries and coats in wet-look gel, scraping it back tight from her forehead into a high ponytail on top of her head, which makes her features look even more harsh than they actually are. She's constantly chewing gum and sneers at people rather than talks to them.

As she taunted Teresa and encouraged her posse to join in with her gibes, I stood at the fence and watched. Teresa tried to ignore them and carry on the game, but when she ran to catch the ball Claire tripped her up and Teresa fell, scraping her chin as she hit the tarmac. It was too much to bear. I grimaced as Teresa hit the ground and felt really bad for her, but

I wanted to escape the painful scene. I walked over to where Mrs. Rose was helping some girl with a twisted ankle and asked to be excused because of severe period pains. I was sent to the nurse's office for some painkillers and a lie-down.

I didn't mention Teresa.

SEVEN

WHEN I GOT HOME AFTER SCHOOL I PHONED EMMA to see how she was and to tell her about the gig on Friday. I didn't know whether to mention Darren or not. We couldn't talk properly on the phone because of my parents anyway. The phone is in the hallway outside the lounge, so they can hear everything. I've been campaigning for my own phone line in my bedroom for years, but Dad says it's as likely to happen as Sadie and Anthony breaking the habit of a lifetime and going on holiday to the moon.

"All right, Leyla, what have you been up to?"

"Sarah and I went to this brilliant gig at the Academy on Friday night: Asian Dub Foundation. It just made me want to be a drummer even more. It's all I want to do, you know."

"Then do it, don't just talk about it. You've got your

drums—all you need to do is keep practicing. You'll be a star before you know it."

"I'm not sure about being a star, but I know I could be a good drummer. I just need to find a band to practice with, that's all. Anyway, how are you? How are you feeling?"

"Oh, you know, okay. Fine most of the time. It gets . . . you know . . . No, I'm fine, I'm fine, honestly."

"Come on, Em, you can talk to me. Don't stop yourself if you want to talk."

"No, really, I'm fine. Listen, there *is* something I wanted to talk to you about, actually. What are you doing now? Can you come down to the flat?"

"Well, I've got some English homework to do for tomorrow, and . . ."

"Tell me about it." Emma groaned. "I am so behind in all of my schoolwork it's not funny. My teachers are on my back about it as well, but I can't exactly turn round and tell them to give me a break because I've just been told I've got HIV and am feeling a bit stressed out lately, can I?"

"Tell them you're having family problems—they always fall for that one. They're well into their stress management these days."

"Oh, I don't know. I just can't seem to concentrate on anything. I haven't been sleeping very well, so I'm knackered half the time, falling asleep at my desk. That's when I'm actually at school and not at the hospital having some test or other done. I've missed so much school it's unbelievable. I'm never going to pass my A Levels next year at this rate."

"Listen, Mum'll have tea ready in a minute, but I can come down at about seven thirty. Shall I ask her if I can stay at your place, and then we can have longer to talk?"

"Yeah, brilliant. See you at seven thirty then," she said, and rang off.

When I arrived at the flat Emma escorted me straight to her room, not giving me a chance to stop and have a quick chat with Aunty Jean, who was sat in the living room watching TV and chain-smoking.

"Did I spot a visitor somewhere in that whirlwind?" she shouted from the couch just as Emma closed her bedroom door firmly behind us.

"I didn't even say hello," I said, catching my breath and struggling to take off my jacket.

"Oh, she's getting on my nerves. I don't want us to end up sitting in the living room with her all night. I thought we could stay in here and chat."

"Fine by me. Get us a drink first, though, will you? I'm gasping."

Emma came bounding back into the room with her arms full of fruit, mineral water, a bag of mixed nuts, and some guacamole dip with tortilla chips. She placed them neatly on the floor at my feet and looked upon her treasure with pride.

"So you're going back to the kitchen for the Coke, chocolate, and crisps then, yeah?' I said, picking up a kiwi fruit, eyeing it suspiciously and wondering what on earth I was going to do with it.

"No way—this is my new healthy eating regime. My doctor has told me that if I pay attention to my diet early on I'm more likely to maintain good health. He's told me all this stuff about how the virus will start to change the structure of my intestines, which means I won't be able to absorb nutrients as well as I would normally, so I've got to get the right balance and correct amount of vitamins and minerals inside me now, to maintain a healthy system and be able to fight off infections."

"Oh, right, I see." I suddenly felt really bad for taking the piss and turning my nose up at her bounty of fresh food. So much had happened, and yet life went on as normal; sometimes I didn't appreciate how much Emma had had to adapt.

"I'll go and buy you a Coke from the corner shop if you want."

"No, no, don't be silly. This cranberry juice looks great to me." I realized how much of an impact HIV was having on every single aspect of her life. Her diet was only one tiny change in the scheme of things that she was having to cope with. But she was just getting on with it.

"A bag of chips or a burger isn't going to kill me or anything," she explained. "They won't do me any harm at all, and the doctor said I shouldn't deprive myself of any treats, but basically I should eat food that is going to give me all the right nutrients so that I stay as healthy as possible. I'm taking loads of vitamin tablets, too. I'm doing quite well so far."

Emma was doing incredibly well. She'd known about being HIV positive for over five months and had coped so well. I'm not with her twenty-four hours a day and she must go through shit when I'm not around to see it, but she's been so brave. I was amazed at how strong and levelheaded she always seems to be. She gets sad and talks about her situation very seriously, but she isn't a total head case; she's holding it together. I'm sure I'd have lost the plot by now if I was her. But you've just got to carry on, haven't you?

Emma spread herself out on some cushions and tucked into the fruit.

"So what's your mum *done* then?" I asked.

"Well, she's got something to do with what I want to talk to you about, actually." She leant over to her bedside table and reached for what looked like her diary. Opening it, she pulled out some A4 sheets and glossy leaflets. "When I was at my counseling session at the clinic last week, my counselor told me about this group in Manchester that is specifically for teenagers who are living with or affected by HIV and AIDS. It's like a support-center kind of thing. Listen, I'll read what it says in the leaflet. 'Positive Living is a self-help center for families living with or affected by HIV and AIDS. We provide support, information, and counseling in a safe and confidential space where families can come and access our services on a weekly basis. We have a teenage group that meets weekly and offers a unique service to those young people who know of their status or that of a family member. Facilitated support sessions allow teenagers the opportunity to share their concerns and discuss issues surrounding HIV and AIDS without fear of judgment or rejection. During the course of the weekly session a range of activities are organized, along with regular trips every month away from the center.' I just wanted you to have a look to see what you think."

I flicked through the different bits of information. There were loads of messages from the teenagers themselves: their experiences of how much the group had helped them to talk about their situation and how it had helped them not to feel so alone because they were with people their own age who understood exactly what was going on in their lives.

"Do you reckon it sounds naff? Like some crappy youth club or something?" Emma asked.

"I dunno, Em. It might be good to meet other kids your age who can understand what you're going through."

"Yeah, I know, but do you reckon I'd end up being dragged round some adventure playground every week or what?" Emma took the leaflets back and studied them again as if looking for some clues, some advice, some hint of what to do for the best.

"You might have to sit around in a circle and hug each other." I giggled.

"Oh God, that's it then. I'm definitely not going." She threw the leaflets across the room.

"No, seriously. Come on, think about it. At the moment only me, your mum, and your counselor know. I just sit around worrying about you half the time, not knowing how to help, and your mum is a wreck. Your counselor sounds brilliant, but she's not exactly the same age as you, is she; she can't know what it's like to be sixteen and have HIV. There'd be people there who could support you properly, who you could make friends with. You might even be able to get some information from them about treatments and all that sort of stuff."

I wasn't sure if I was being selfish, but I was relieved to find out there was a group out there that might be able to help Em, because I often felt inadequate to help her or to know what she was going through.

"I'm just a bit . . . you know . . . scared. I mean, I don't know what the other kids are going to be like. What if I don't get on with them? And I don't think I'm ready to open up to a bunch of complete strangers about what's happened to me anyway. Besides, *she* isn't too happy about it." Emma cocked her head in the direction of the living room. "The counselor told her that it would be a really good idea if she went along to the parents' group at the same time because it would be an opportunity for her to talk and get some help and information. She hasn't got anyone to confide in: Nan is dead. Dad . . . well, he hasn't been sighted for years. And it's not as though she's very close to your mum—they barely have a civil word to say to each other. But she's being a stubborn old bag and said she won't go near the place. She doesn't want anyone knowing her private business or telling her how to look after her daughter. She says that she can cope fine on her own and doesn't need anybody interfering in our lives."

"But what about you, though? Is she going to stop you going as well?"

"Well, I don't think she'll stop me, but she is worried about me talking to so many people about my illness and it eventually getting back to someone around here and ruining my life. It's her pride, too, you know. She wants to feel as though I can always rely on her for a shoulder to cry on. She finds the fact that I go to a counselor difficult enough as it is, but the thought of me sharing things with a whole group of people freaks her out a bit, I guess. She won't even look at the leaflets.

"Anyway, I don't care what she thinks. I'm going to go if I decide to, and she'll just have to handle it. It's my life." Emma got to her feet and started tidying things up in her room while I leant over to her stereo to put on a CD.

"You could come with me," she announced suddenly as if she'd just struck upon the best idea in the world. "If I started going, that is." She plonked herself back down on the cushions and looked straight at me with a pleading expression. "I'd just feel so much more comfortable if you were there as well. You understand what I've been going through, you've been there all the way practically, and I'm sure they wouldn't mind you coming along as someone to support me."

I was a bit taken aback. I could understand her wanting some company—it's horrible joining any sort of group for the first time on your own. But it didn't feel right. "Oh, Em, I don't know. I'll think about it. But perhaps it would be better to go on your own. You'll make new friends straightaway. It'll be a bit scary the first time you go but after that it'll be fine. You won't rely on me so much if I'm not there, and you'll probably talk more and get more out of the group, because you'll be forced to join in."

Em folded her arms behind her head and lay back on the floor, staring up at the ceiling. "Yeah, you're probably right. Mum has just unsettled my nerves by being so negative and paranoid about the whole thing. My confidence is a bit low at the moment, that's all."

"So do you reckon you're going to go then?"

"I'm not sure. I'll think about it this week."

We got into our pajamas and sat snuggled up in her double bed together, then talked for ages about school and friends and everything really. I feel as though I can talk to Emma about anything in the world. We played some CDs and talked about music and I got all revved up about being in a band one day and found myself rambling on about my future career as a rock legend.

Emma had pulled out some photos of us on my first day at secondary school five years ago. We were stood outside my house. Emma was four feet off the ground, jumping into the air behind me as I stood with hunched shoulders and stared down in horror at my awful brown Clarks with their sensible cork soles. Emma refused to bend to convention, even at the age of eleven, and had customized her uniform with a silk scarf around her neck and a pink glitter belt around her waist.

Not a single hair was out of place on my head and I was wearing regulation everything: knee-length socks that had been bleached for extra whiteness, a starched A-line skirt, and the best regulation navy blue school jumper money could buy. My mum had insisted on me looking immaculate. "You're not showing this family up," she'd warned.

"'The best years of your life' is what they say about school, you know," Emma said softly, not taking her eyes off the photo and letting a few tears drop from her nose.

After school on Thursday, Emma was waiting for me outside the gates. I was on my own because Sarah was staying late for some meeting or other, so I was glad to see Em and relieved not to have to go straight home.

"Let's go to Georgio's for a chat. If we can actually manage to get any privacy there, that is," Emma said.

Georgio's is the café on the high street where everyone from our school hangs out. It's nothing special; it's just your regular greasy spoon. The only reason everyone goes there is because Georgio and the rest of his Greek family who run it don't seem to mind a table of five schoolkids huddling around one cup of coffee between them. Occasionally someone will buy a cheese sandwich and a cheer will go up for the last of the big spenders.

Tucked away right at the back of the café next to the toilets is a booth with high-backed red leather seats, and that's where everyone goes to have a sneaky fag. When you look in from the street you can't actually see who is sat in the booth; there's just a cloud of smoke hovering above whoever's sat there. Different cliques of friends have their own tables. Some groups have even gone so far as to scratch their names into the Formica tabletops to mark out their territory. Every weekday you can guarantee that there will be someone from our school in there. I've never walked past without seeing a splash of navy blue uniform. Sometimes on my way to school at eight thirty in the morning I see gangs of girls already sipping cappuccinos for their breakfast, chins wagging as though they've never left from the night before.

It's a different story on the weekend, though. On Saturdays you couldn't get a seat if you tried. It's chocker-full of grannies blocking the aisles with their shopping trolleys, and mothers with their children and pushchairs. You can guarantee that they'd all sat in exactly the same seats years ago when they were at school themselves, and I often prayed that I wouldn't be going to the same caff a few years down the line with a bunch of screaming kids round my ankles, scrabbling the money together for a cup of tea.

Emma and I managed to get a corner table by ourselves and ordered a Coke with two straws.

"I've spoken to someone at the support center," Emma said with slightly more enthusiasm than at the beginning of the week.

"What did they say? Are you going to go?"

"Well, yeah, they want me to go along this Saturday to have a look around, meet some people, and just have a chat with them. I don't have to keep going if I don't like it."

"Are you still worried about going on your own, though?"

"No, no, not really. I mean, of course I'm nervous about the whole thing, but, well, they sounded really nice on the phone."

"What does your mum think? Have you told her they've invited you there on Saturday?"

"She's come round to the idea a little bit, and she's given

her consent, but she's still adamant that she doesn't want to have anything to do with it herself. My counselor says she's still trying to come to terms with my illness, that she's a long way from accepting what has happened to me and that that's why she's rejecting help and support. She can't seem to see that by going to this center they would be able to help her come to terms with what has happened and to move on. Anyway, she's said that she'll come into Manchester with me, take me to the center to check out what sort of place it is, and will come back at the end of the day to pick me up. She keeps saying that she won't be staying very long, but we'll see."

"I hope it's all right. It's worth having a look, anyway, and as you say, if it's too much like being back in the Brownies you can just walk."

"Well, watch this space. What are *you* up to on the weekend?"

"Me and Sarah have been invited to a party that somebody from school is having at a new bar in town on Saturday night. Why don't you come after you get back from the center—you can tell me all about it then. It should be a good night. Good music, I reckon. I know the DJ."

"Yeah, I'd love to. I feel as though I haven't been out partying for ages. Then again, I haven't exactly had much to celebrate. Just let me know all the details and I'll meet you there. Who's this DJ then? Anyone I know?" she quizzed me.

"Oh no, just some boy I met at that gig the other night. He's in our sixth form; name's Darren. He seems to have okay taste in music, so he should play some decent stuff."

"I could do with a good night out."

"Listen, I'd better go. Mum'll have the tea on, and you know what she's like if I'm late and disrupt the timetable."

"You'd better get yourself home and report for duty then." Emma grabbed me by the arm and frog-marched me out of Georgio's in exaggerated military style: "Left, right, left, right, left, right."

I woke up early on Saturday morning thinking about the party. I couldn't seem to get Darren out of my head; I was really looking forward to seeing him again. It was crazy, because I didn't even know him properly. All I knew was that he was gorgeous and had the most beautiful to-die-for eyes. He seemed more mature than the other guys I knew—at least he hadn't talked nonstop about fast cars and football in front of me. And the best thing was that he loved music and knew his stuff. I was sure we could spend hours bending each other's ears about the latest samplers and drum machines. It was quite clear to me that we were made for each other.

Sarah and I had planned that I'd get to her house at about seven o'clock to get ready. Her mum goes to her church every Saturday to clear up the confetti after a wedding and to make sure the place is spick-and-span for the Sunday service. Afterward she goes for tea with the priest. It's great, because we get to have the house to ourselves. We can turn up the music and have plenty of space to get ready in.

But it seemed that seven o'clock would never come, so I just lay down on the fluffy rug in my room and flicked through some magazines and let my mind drift. I started thinking about Sarah's mum and all that religion stuff again. I don't think I'm religious or anything. Well, I've never really been to church apart from school carol services at Christmas, so I don't know much about it all, but sometimes I can't help thinking that if there is a God why does he or she allow such terrible things like HIV to happen to people? Why are there so many natural disasters in this world and so many diseases, wars, and murders? What answer could Sarah's mum give me? If God is so powerful and so good, why doesn't he or she install love and peace forever and ever, amen?

I know it's not that simple and I realize that the world is of our own making, but with things like HIV, which seem to be completely beyond any human being's control, it just makes you wonder why these things happen in the first place. What's it all about, you know? It gets you thinking, but if you think too much about it you just end up going round and round in circles. I don't think anyone knows the answer, not really. All I know is that a lot of bad things and a lot of good things happen in life and at the end of the day you've just got to get on with it.

I realized that I had been lying on my bedroom floor letting thoughts whirl around the room and bounce off the walls for quite some time. It was catching sight of my leopard-print top with the slashed neck poking out of my wardrobe that made me think about the party again. I'd decided to wear it with a pair of black trousers and my new sneakers, all set off by my cute pink choker with the tiny diamond studs. I wondered whether my diamanté tiara was going too far—I wasn't really sure what sort of a party it was going to be. I started getting a bit nervous thinking about Darren. Why had he invited us in the first place? Did he like me? I was worried that it would be awkward when I saw him because I hadn't seen him since he turned up at Sarah and my den at school, and I didn't even know if he'd remember inviting us. I was so glad that Sarah was going with me. She'll talk to anyone, even if it's only to give out abuse.

My stomach rumbled. I hadn't eaten since breakfast, so I

went downstairs to make myself a sandwich. Mum was in the kitchen ironing and Sadie was sat at the table painting her nails.

"Oh, so you've deigned to join us at last. What have you been doing?" Mum asked.

"Oh, just philosophizing about religion, relationships, whether one wears a tiara to parties in Bury or not. You know, just your regular teenage musings on a Saturday afternoon."

"You're a cocky little madam sometimes." Mum looked disapprovingly in my direction as I squeezed behind her and the ironing board to get to the fridge.

"Whose party are you going to?" Sadie said without looking up from her polished nails.

"One of Sarah's friends is having a birthday party," I lied. Mum thinks Sarah is such a good-mannered, well-brought-up girl that she trusts me to do anything if she's involved. She's always going on about Sarah's disciplined, religious upbringing and wishes I were as well behaved as her. It makes me laugh—how wrong can parents be?—but I'm not going to correct her.

"So are you wearing the tiara or not?" Sadie quizzed.

"What on earth do you want to go wearing a tiara for? You'll just draw attention to yourself, have a swarm of young men buzzing around you and getting you into trouble," Mum said, waving the iron at me.

"Why do girls always get the blame for attracting attention to themselves when they get hassled by blokes just because they've got nice clothes on that they like wearing and that make them feel good about themselves? I'm making a fashion statement, not trying to impress the lads."

"I've seen girls downtown going out looking like floozies,

with skirts that look more like belts and tops that show off all of their cleavage. They're asking for trouble," Mum retorted.

"So, do you reckon all women should walk around in sacks to stop men from being led into temptation? Why can't blokes just have some respect for girls no matter what they're wearing?"

"You might think you know it all, young lady, but believe you me it's a wicked world and things aren't as simple as you might think. If I ever see you out on the streets dressed like . . . like a . . . a hussy, I'll have your guts for garters." By now, Mum was ironing at a furious pace, her face all red as though she was going to blow up in a puff of hot steam.

I couldn't be bothered to argue. Mum always draws any argument back to the fact that she is older and wiser and she knows best, and that I'm just young and naïve and I'll learn from experience eventually.

In my haste to get out of the kitchen and as far away from Mum and Sadie as possible, I barged past the kitchen table, knocking over Sadie's nail polish as I went.

"Oh, Leyla, now look what you've done," Sadie screeched.

"So what? You're only drawing attention to yourself wearing that sleazy nail polish anyway. Imagine all the trouble you could get into." I smiled sarcastically in Mum's direction and skipped out of the kitchen.

The party was in the upstairs room of what used to be Valentino's wine bar, the sort of cheesy disco that Sadie goes to for a night out with the girls from Abbey National. It's just been bought out by some trendy Manchester club owner who's got plans for revamping it and getting some big-name DJs in there. He's named it the Mars Bar.

We walked into the downstairs bar, sticking to the carpet,

looking for the stairs, and were pushed out of the way by a gang of girls on a hen night running after a distressed bride-to-be who had just caught her fiancé snogging someone in the Ladies. It was still Valentino's wine bar, new owner or not. The only difference was a precarious vase of fancy flowers on top of the jukebox and a list of posh beers chalked up on the blackboard and a sign advertising bowls of olives for £2.50. Despite those few minor changes, I still expected to see Sadie sipping a Bacardi Breezer in the corner.

Upstairs at the party, Sarah and I skirted around the periphery of the dance floor and tried to suss out who we knew there. Sarah spotted one of her brother Jamie's friends, so we went over to speak to him. It was mostly an older crowd of kids from sixth form and the local colleges, so I felt a bit self-conscious about being much younger than everyone else. I began to wish that I hadn't worn my tiara after all, despite Sarah's telling me a thousand times how fantastic I looked.

While Sarah chewed the ear off her newfound friend, I had time to search the room for Darren. I couldn't see him anywhere and was beginning to feel a little disappointed, thinking that he might not even show up, when I spotted him in the DJ booth with his headphones on, head down, concentrating on his decks like he was doing a maths test. I felt too shy to go up to him straightaway. I had a few butterflies in my stomach and wasn't sure what to say to him. I kept glancing at him out of the corner of my eye while trying to get in on the conversation Sarah was having, because I didn't want to be just stood around staring at him like a complete idiot. Eventually he stopped concentrating on his decks and caught me looking at him. Our eyes locked. He waved me over and I walked nervously toward the DJ box.

"All right? How long have you been here?" he asked.

"Oh, we've only just arrived. Enough time for Sarah to corner some bloke who will soon wish he'd never left the house tonight."

"Yeah, she's a feisty lady, that's for sure."

"Oh, she's great. I love her to bits. She's just got a gob on her like the Mersey tunnel, that's all."

"Well, anyway, welcome to the salubrious setting of Darren Mitchell's disco inferno," he said, twirling around in the tiny space.

"What are you putting on next?"

"I don't know. Why don't you choose. Surprise me."

I knelt down at his silver chrome record boxes, crammed full of vinyl, and started flicking through his collection. I was glad I had a chance to take a deep breath and try to calm myself down a bit. I wanted him to like me, but if I carried on being such a nervous wreck he was just going to think I was a dizzy idiot. I pulled out one of Sarah and my all-time-favorite tracks, one that I knew she would go mad for when she heard it. I removed it from the sleeve so Darren wouldn't know what it was and gestured for him to move out of the way so I could put it on.

"Do you know what to do?" he asked, looking a little anxious.

"Well, I've only ever used my gran's gramophone, but I'm sure I'll find my way around this new contraption," I said, totally deadpan, and when I was sure he was suitably worried I cracked a smile and punched his arm playfully. "Of course I know how to operate decks, for God's sake. You're not one of those blokes who think that boys spin the discs and girls flaunt themselves on the podium, are you?"

"No, of course not. I'd just forgotten you're as much of an anorak as I am."

"I'll take that as a compliment, shall I?"

Sarah went ballistic when our tune came on and dragged me away from the DJ box to dance. I felt great. It hadn't been so awkward talking to Darren after all, and he had seemed genuinely pleased to see me. I spent the rest of the night between the dance floor and Darren, and at about ten thirty Emma showed up. She'd got a taxi from her house, having dropped her mum off after they got back from the support center. We sneaked off to a quiet corner so I could fire questions at her about her day: "How was it? What were the people like? Was it a nice place? What did you do?"

"Leyla, I don't know where to start. It was mind-blowing. I was terrified walking into the room for the first time, thinking that all eyes were going to be on me—the positive one. But when I realized that it was a room full of people just like me who either had HIV or knew someone in their family who had it . . ." Emma gulped and fought back tears. "Oh God, I don't know, it made me want to cry with relief. Just seeing people my age, knowing that they understood what was happening to me, was incredible. All the times I've been to the clinic in Manchester for tests or whatever, I've never seen anyone my age, or even another girl, come to think of it. It's bound to make you feel like a freak after a while."

"Oh, Em, I'm so glad it worked out okay. I've been thinking about you all day."

"I mean, I felt a bit weird because it was like really facing up to the fact that I'm . . ." Emma looked around to check that nobody was in earshot and dropped her voice to barely a whisper. ". . . that I'm HIV positive, you know. It really brought it home to me. I was freaked out when I went to the center because the first woman I saw looked really, really ill and it scared the hell out of me. I suddenly felt that I didn't belong there. I'm not ill; I don't look ill. I felt like a fake or something. I just wanted to run home and watch Saturday morning TV like everyone else and forget any of it was happening, but luckily I was ushered into the youth center, where everyone was just sat around watching telly, listening to music, and gossiping, and that calmed me down a bit."

"Was everyone in the youth center talking about being HIV positive and stuff?"

"No, not really. Before I even went into the main center itself, Lucinda, one of the coordinators of the center, took me and my mum into this room and just had a quick chat with us. She told me that everyone in the group was affected by HIV and AIDS one way or another. She explained that some of the teenagers were HIV positive while others had parents or siblings who were positive or who had died of AIDS-related causes. So even though nobody was talking about HIV outright today, there was an understanding that everyone knew why they were there. That was what was so amazing about it all for me. I hadn't actually talked to anyone else with HIV before today, Leyla. I've been sat in that flat thinking that I must be the only sixteen-year-old girl in the whole world with it."

I was in awe of what Emma had to say. It must have been awful for her all those months not knowing another person who was in the same boat as her. I wanted to hear more.

"What did you do all day?" I asked.

"We just hung out really. You know: We had dinner, played CDs, mucked around on the PlayStation and the computer. I made you something, actually. I was just playing around with the clip art on the computer. It's silly really." Emma pulled a folded piece of A4 paper out of her jacket pocket and passed it to me. It was a picture of a big red heart with sparkly stars all around it, and in the middle it said: "Thank you for being my best mate. You're a star. Love, Em."

"Oh, Em, it's beautiful. Thank you. I'm really touched. It's gorgeous."

"It's nothing. I was just fiddling around. It could have been better but we had to stop everything we were doing at one point to get together and have this big talk. Everyone's supposed to talk about how they're feeling, what they've been doing, any points they'd like to raise about the group, and stuff like that. Not everyone spoke, though, and I just about managed to tell everyone my name."

"Did you have a group hug?" I giggled.

"Nah, it wasn't like that at all. It was dead normal."

"How's your mum?"

"She's okay. She stayed for the minimum amount of time she could get away with and headed straight out of the door as soon as possible."

"So you going back then?"

"Definitely. I mean, I was really shy and scared, but it showed me that I'm not on my own."

We were both quietly thinking about everything Em had just said when Sarah came bounding over to us, leapt on my back, and demanded to know why we were huddled together, acting all secretive. "What are you two boring old wallflowers up to? You're cooking something up, aren't you? Come on, tell me. What's with all this hiding in corners?"

"It's nothing, we're just chatting," I told her. "Catching up, discussing who's here, who's not, and planning how we can help that poor boy you've been draped over all night to make his escape."

"Oh, very funny. I'll have you know he's been attached to my side like a limpet all night. It's me who wants to get rid of him, thank you. He's got Lynx aftershave on. I mean, purrleese, as if I'm going to be interested in anyone who's wearing anything less than Calvin Klein."

I felt bad for Emma, because I knew she hated having to hide so much from people, especially those she cared about, but there didn't seem to be any choice. It was something we *both* had to cope with: I hated keeping anything from Sarah, but I didn't know what else to do.

We headed over to the dance floor, and Emma got to chatting with some people she knew and slotted into the crowd like the missing piece of a jigsaw puzzle. That's what Emma is like. She just seems to fit in wherever she goes, whatever she does, with no effort. She breezes into any social situation and makes it look easy. People really gravitate to her, because she makes everyone feel so relaxed and comfortable. I wish I was more like her sometimes. I tend to stand back and observe and worry about what people are thinking, and live inside my head a lot, instead of just launching into a situation and living it there and then.

Darren had finished his DJing slot and was slowly making his way over to us. "Hello there, disco divas." Sarah rolled her eyes and resumed her position on Mr. Lynx aftershave's hip.

"Is this your DJ friend?" Emma asked.

Darren took her hand, twirled her around, and, bringing her to his chest, said, "DJ Darren, that's my name. Whatever the mood, whatever the occasion, I've got the disc to make you twist." Emma pulled herself away and laughed.

"This is my cousin Emma. God, you're a cheese ball."

"I know," he said, laughing at himself.

Darren makes me laugh. I know Sarah thinks he's a show-off, but he's more of a show*man* than a show-*off*, I reckon.

We joked around and danced for a while, until the clock struck midnight and I had to get home before my carriage turned into a pumpkin and my clothes turned to rags. I'd asked Mum if Emma and Sarah could come back to our place and stay the night, and she'd said okay, so we called a cab and waited by the door for it to turn up. When it eventually arrived, Darren walked with us out onto the street and opened the cab door for us to get in.

"You'll be putting your coat over a puddle for us next," Sarah said sarcastically.

"Can't a boy be chivalrous nowadays without getting his head snapped off?" Darren replied, sticking his head inside the car to confront Sarah.

"Chivalry gives me the shivers," Sarah retorted. She folded her arms across her chest and stared straight ahead, obviously not prepared to talk about it further.

"Well, adios. See you later." Darren bent down, kissed me on my cheek, and shut the door firmly.

I was smitten.

"That boy is so slimy, Leyla, I don't know what you see in him. He loves himself so badly," Sarah said, exasperated with me.

"So what's the deal with you two then? Are you, like, seeing each other properly or what? I can't believe you haven't told me about him." Emma nudged me in the ribs and squeezed my knee, demanding answers.

"Nothing's going on. That's only the third time I've ever spoken to him in my life. I met him at the Academy at that gig I told you about. He goes to our school. He invited me and

Sarah along tonight, and we get on really well. That's all there is to know. There's nothing going on. I can't believe he actually kissed me good-bye. We barely know each other."

I must have looked pretty doe-eyed and smitten, because Sarah was suddenly shoving her fingers down her throat, making gagging noises and asking me to pass the bucket.

"Right. For that you're sleeping on the floor tonight, missy, and if you give me any more grief I'll make you sleep in the spare bed in Sadie's room," I threatened. "And you know she's got pictures of Posh and Becks all over her walls that will give you nightmares you'll never forget."

"Okay, okay, I'll behave, I'll behave. I've only got your best interests at heart, though, Leyla. I just think you're too special to waste your time on plonkers who love themselves too much, that's all."

I was reading a book in my room the following Saturday night when Emma called round the house. It was about nine o'clock. She'd just come back from another day at the support center. "I didn't expect to see you here tonight. Is everything okay?" I asked.

"Of course it is. I'm not always the purveyor of doom, you know."

"I didn't mean it like that. I'm just surprised to see you."

"So was your mum. And she was upset that I'd caught her in her ski pants and slippers and kept apologizing for the state of the place. What's she like? This house is a palace."

"I wish she'd stop caring about appearances and what other people think all the time and just concentrate on the more important things in life."

"Like drumming, you mean?"

"Yeah, that's right, like drumming. Are you taking the piss?"

"No, honestly I'm not. I came round specifically to *talk* to you about drumming, actually."

"Oh yeah? Sounds ominous. Go on." I eyed Emma suspiciously, wondering what she was getting at.

"Well, today at the center we were talking about all the different things we're going to be doing with the group over the next few weeks. There's trips to the bowling alley and the flicks and a few meals organized—you know the sort of thing. Anyway, some people suggested that they'd like to set up a music workshop—have music lessons and try and put some music together or something like that. Lucinda said that we might be able to use the music college in Salford as a base, because apparently they're really good about letting the center make use of their equipment and facilities. But first of all we need to find people who can come in and help run the workshops. You know, musicians to teach new skills and help with composing some music."

"God, you really are getting involved now, aren't you?" I said, pleased. "I knew it would take you about five minutes to settle in there."

"I wasn't so nervous today, but I still feel a bit awkward and shy there. I'm becoming so used to hiding my status like it doesn't really exist that it's weird getting used to the fact that I'm surrounded by people who aren't going to judge me or walk away from me like I'm a piece of dirt."

'Plus, I bet you can't actually believe why you're there in the first place."

"Yeah, it's that and all. But at least I am trying to face up to it, which is more than my mum is doing."

"So, have you made any friends yet or what?"

"There's a couple of girls who seem quite nice whom I

talked to a bit. There's Shula; she's been going for a couple of years but seems as on edge and shy as I am when I'm there. We're the ones who hang back and try to make ourselves look as small and as inconspicuous as possible. I think we saw an ally in each other today, so we ended up chatting nervously later on. And there's Ellie, who is a bit sort of, umm, quirky, I suppose—quite odd really. She just came bounding up to me today and started telling me all about her mum, who used to be a really popular singer in Canada before she got ill, and how she wanted to sing and follow in her mum's footsteps if the music workshop came off. She made me feel more relaxed because she was so mad."

"So why do you want to talk to me about drumming then?"

"I thought you could teach people the drums." I sat up straight at that point and asked her exactly what she meant. "Well, I told them that my cousin was a top-class drummer who would be happy to share her skills with others."

"Emma, I am not a musician. I couldn't teach anyone else how to play, let alone compose a piece of music. Not if I were paid a million pounds."

"That's another thing: It would be voluntary. They haven't got enough money to pay anyone, so they're relying on people's goodwill. I told them you had plenty of that."

"Hold on a minute. Are you listening to me? I wouldn't know how to teach anyone the drums. I'm only learning myself."

"Oh, you're too modest for your own good. You're a brilliant drummer. You'd easily be able to teach people a few basic skills. Will you do it or not?"

"Are you just doing this so that you'll have me for company at the center, because if you are . . ."

"I'm not. I'm not," Emma protested. "The workshop would only be every other Saturday, so you wouldn't be there with me every week. I've got to get used to the place sooner or later."

"Oh, Em, I dunno. I'm not sure I could handle it, like."

I was stumbling over my words. I couldn't really express my worries exactly, but the thought of going to the center, where people were ill, or where I could even catch something myself, made me feel very uneasy. I realized that my prejudices were becoming apparent. "I'd feel like the odd one out," were the words that came spilling unexpectedly from my mouth.

"Why? Because you'd be the only one not dying or something?" Emma looked hurt.

A heavy tension immediately followed. I felt the blood slowly creep up my neck and burst into my face. I was flustered and nervous. We fidgeted and looked away from each other. I wished that the conversation had never happened. I felt so bad. I was letting Emma down. I was frightened and shocked by the workings of my own mind. It was as though I had learnt to cope with Em's status, but when it came to pushing the boundaries any further I was paralyzed by my fears.

And yet all she was asking of me was to help out with a music workshop. I knew how much Emma needed to make things around her as normal as possible, and perhaps I could bring some normality to the unfamiliar world that she'd entered at the center. Just stopping to think about what Emma was actually going through made me realize that if I was scared, then Emma must be petrified out of her wits living with a disease like HIV every day of her life, not knowing if she's going to fall ill suddenly, not knowing how long she has to live. It made me shudder to think about it, and I knew I had to get a grip on myself. I had to be strong.

"Em, I'm sorry. I'll do it. I'll do it. Will there be other people helping out as well, though?"

Emma smiled, but still looked sad and distant. "Of course there'll be others. I think they already know a singer and a guitarist. I don't want us to fall out over any of this, though, Leyla. I shouldn't have pressurized you so much. Come if you want to, but I don't want to force you."

"It's all right, I'm just being silly. It'll be fine. Anything for you."

"No, no, it's all in the name of music, remember," she teased, knowing that at the end of the day I would love the opportunity to get out of the garage and play with some real musicians. "Listen, I'd better go. It's getting late and Mum will be wondering where I am." Em hopped off the bed and gathered up her stuff.

As we walked past the living room, we popped our heads round the door; Emma thought it was only polite to say goodbye to the oldies. Mum and Dad were both fast asleep on the sofa, with their slippers kicked off in front of them. Dad was snoring loudly. There were half-eaten nibbles in little bowls on the coffee table next to an empty Blockbuster video case. The film played unnoticed in the corner. They'd probably only managed to stay awake for the opening scene. It was always the same. I rolled my eyes at Emma and saw her to the door.

"See you sometime next week," I said, waving her off down the road.

Now that I was alone and relieved to have smoothed over any bad feeling with Em, I realized that I was in fact quite fired up at the prospect of doing these drum workshops. For quite a while I had been thinking how good it would be to actually play with some other musicians and attempt for the first time ever to put some music together, and now was my chance. I was scared but pretty excited, all at the same time. I just hoped that I'd be good enough and that I wouldn't let Emma down. It's one thing mucking around in a garage on your own and quite another teaching people and putting your skills to the test. I suddenly panicked that I couldn't really play the drums at all, and felt that I had to get on them just to calm myself down.

It was gone ten o'clock and I was banned from stepping foot in the garage after eight, but hearing Dad's snores get louder and louder, I thought I could sneak in for a quick bash before Mum woke up with a stiff neck and pinched Dad awake to tell him he was missing half the film.

I lit the candles in the garage as I liked to do at night to create a bit of an atmosphere, then put the gas heater on. I slid my headphones on, pressed play on my CD player, and started drumming softly but deliberately along to the music blaring from my headphones. I thought I was being quiet, but I must have got carried away and worked my way up to a crescendo, because the main lights suddenly went on and I saw Mum, Dad, Sadie, and Anthony stood at the door with their arms crossed and lips pursed, staring right at me. I realized I'd gotten so involved I had broken into a sweat.

Sadie, who had just got back from the Bull and Gate with her worse half, began things as I reached down to turn my CD off. "Anthony and I could hear your racket before we even turned the corner into the estate, couldn't we, Anthony?"

Anthony, who had obviously had one shandy too many, was swaying on the step leading down to the garage, but nodded on cue as though Sadie had pulled a few strings at the back of his neck. He is such a dummy, I thought.

Mum was next. "You've spoilt your father and my Saturday night. We hired a video as a treat, only to have it ruined by this commotion. We couldn't hear ourselves think in there. What do you think you're playing at? You've got no respect or consideration for anyone." Mum was positively boiling over with rage. The veins on her temples were standing out and spit was flying everywhere as she lashed out at me. "What the hell do you think you're doing at this time of the night?" she said, moving her hands to rest on her hips so that I knew she meant business.

I stared back at all four of them, thinking how ridiculous they all looked. Dad with his shirt half in and half out of his trousers, scratching his ruffled bedhead, barely awake enough to know what all the fuss was about. Mum in her ski pants and socked feet stuffed inside pink fluffy mules, itching for a fight. And Anthony, who was ready to collapse into a drunken sleep, propped up by my smug older sister, who loved nothing more than seeing me get into trouble.

I couldn't be bothered to waste my breath trying to excuse myself. I had one last loud and furious turn on my drums before throwing my sticks down and barging past the whole lot of them back to my bedroom. Anthony fell off the step as I marched by, and I heard Sadie tut and tell him to get a grip on himself.

They all made me laugh. What a bunch of total losers. I threw myself onto my bed and wished I could be anywhere in the world but 30 Beech Glen. What the hell did they know about music and ambition? They'll be sorry when I'm rich and famous, I told myself. I'll be more than happy to remind them of the total lack of support and enthusiasm they showed me. They're far too worried about what the neighbors will think and not having their TV viewing interrupted to care that a musical genius is blossoming under their noses. I stuck my head farther beneath the duvet and tried to block out my surroundings before sinking into an exhausted sleep.

The next day I woke up late, and could sense the frosty atmosphere in the house even before I'd stepped out of my room. I could hear Mum slamming things around in the kitchen and giving Sadie monosyllabic answers to her questions. I couldn't believe that Mum was still so angry with me. Anyone would have thought I'd committed murder the night before. For a fraction of a second I thought that maybe I should apologize and make peace, if only for a quiet life, but I soon got over that and decided to carry on as normal as though nothing had happened.

I knew this would infuriate Mum further, but I just couldn't be bothered to suck up to her. Mum and Dad never show any interest in what I do and treat me like a freak for spending so much time on my drums on my own. They've never tried to understand what I'm attempting to achieve. Okay, so drums aren't the most sociable of instruments, but they're my passion. The way they tried to control and suppress what they called "just a phase" made me want to bash around on my drums at three o'clock every sodding morning.

I decided to brave the wintry climate in the kitchen and breezed in with a smile, full of the joys of spring. Mum, who had turned into the Ice Queen of Narnia, glared at me from the sink.

"You can take that smile off your face. Your behavior last

night was unforgivable. You displayed a total lack of respect and consideration for me and your father, not to mention the neighbors, and we will not tolerate it. You know the rules, Leyla. We expect an apology from you."

She stood calm and upright at the sink waiting for my pleas for forgiveness, but I couldn't take her seriously, as her yellow marigold gloves and pale blue overalls failed to convey any air of authority. I kept thinking of our school dinner ladies and lumpy custard and found it hard to suppress a smirk. "Right. That's it! The garage door will remain locked until you decide to show some respect."

"That's not fair. You're treating me like a criminal just for having a quick practice on my drums. Do you want me to achieve anything in this life or not?"

"You won't achieve anything without discipline and respect for others, Leyla, and the sooner you learn that lesson the better."

"How about *you* showing *me* some respect for once? Okay, so maybe I shouldn't have been playing quite so loudly at that time of night. I got a bit carried away. But the way you treat me for playing the drums at all is totally unreasonable. You just don't seem to care that music means a lot to me. It's what I want to do with my life. Why can't you take me seriously and give me some support?"

A tense, heavy silence followed as Mum and I stood looking at each other across the kitchen. Sadie was sat at the table with her mouth wide open, lapping it all up as if it were an episode of *EastEnders*. For a moment it seemed that Mum and I were desperate to understand each other but that neither of us knew where to start. Mum turned back to the sink and carried on with the washing up, muttering that the garage was off limits until Dad and her received an apology.

I couldn't bear to stay in the house any longer, so I threw on my coat and headed out the door in the direction of Sarah's. I ran down the road and out of the estate, glad to be in the open air and away from the house. I needed some space, and the fresh breeze cooled me down. I knew that I'd have to grit my teeth and tread carefully with Mum for a while in order to get my garage privileges back, but I felt so frustrated with her. I just wanted to break free of her for the day and think about something and someone completely different. I knew that Sarah's company would be the perfect cure.

"All right, missy. What a pleasant surprise to see your grumpy old face on this fine Sunday morning." Sarah was her usual self as she opened the door to me.

"Do I look grumpy?" I asked, surprised.

"You've got a face like a slapped arse."

"Sorry. It's just Mum, you know. Listen, forget it. I don't want to talk about her. Cheer me up, Sarah."

"Well, actually, despite my better judgment I might have some news that will put a smile on your face."

I perked up immediately and followed Sarah to her room. "Go on then. What is it?"

"Have I shown you the new nail varnish I bought last week? It's a wicked color. I thought it would go with my sparkly pink top," Sarah teased as she browsed over the cosmetics on her dressing table.

"Sarah, don't be such a witch. Tell me the news."

"Oh, it's not that exciting really. You won't be interested."

"Sarah, I'm gonna kill you." I pulled her onto the bed and sat on top of her chest, pinning her down. "Tell me the news."

"Okay, okay, okay, get off me,' she said, struggling. "I'm

flat-chested enough as it is without you making it any worse."

"Do you promise to tell me?"

"Yes, yes. Now get off me." I jumped off and she sat up straight at the end of the bed, all smugness because she knew something she knew I'd be interested in. "Jamie told me this morning that he's going to watch a skateboarding competition down at the park at midday with a bunch of his mates. Apparently it's the regional championships and a lad from our school is tipped to win because he's won most of the local competitions all year."

"Is that it? Some kids skidding around on boards and that's news?"

"Oh, I just thought you might like to know that the local champion is in fact Darren Mitchell. Loverboy himself. *Your* Darren." Sarah turned her back to me and pretended to be engrossed in the contents of a shampoo bottle on her dressing table. "But if you're not interested in a bunch of kids 'skidding around on boards' then don't worry, we'll just stay in and watch telly instead."

"What do you mean, *my* Darren?" I asked, blushing.

"Oh come on, don't go all coy on me. You've hardly been subtle about how much you like him. Hanging around the corridors after every lesson hoping to catch a glimpse of him. Holding your breath every time someone walks past our secret place just in case it's him coming to see you. You're so transparent, Miss Burgess. You can't hide a thing from me."

"I thought I was playing it really cool." We both fell about laughing at how blatant I'd been. "So he's a champion skate-boarder as well as a totally gorgeous, talented DJ. But why would you want to point out another of his many assets to me when you can't stand him?"

"Well, you're my best mate, and call me a softy, but I thought that seeing as you haven't managed to get a fix of him at school all this week, you might need one—and soon."

Without a moment's hesitation, I grabbed my coat. "I love you. Let's go." I jumped up, kissed Sarah on the forehead, and was practically out of the door before she had time to put her shoes on. But I stopped sharp before I got outside.

"Hold on—do I look all right? What if he thinks I'm stalking him? He's not going to want to talk to me on his big day. He probably won't even remember me. This is stupid. My hair's a mess. We'll just go and hang around at the back of the crowd, okay? We'll check it out from a distance." Sarah stood at the front door staring at me like I was mad. "What's up?" I asked.

"You're unbelievable. Calm down. You look great, and we'll just go and hang out for a while. See what happens, okay?"

When we got down to the park I was relieved to see that gathered around the skateboard ramps was quite a big crowd that I could easily get lost in. Gangs of cute-looking boys with goatees, wearing big baggy skatewear and benny hats, were stood around comparing one another's Day-Glo motifs on the bottoms of their boards. We spotted Jamie and his mates and went over to them. I just wanted to see Darren once and told myself I'd be satisfied with that. Jamie must have been talking to me, because the next thing I knew Sarah was kicking my foot to try to get my attention and explaining to Jamie that I had a crush on some sixth-former and wasn't worth talking to because he wouldn't get any decent conversation out of me.

I started to think that I was turning into a bit of a loser

spending so much time thinking about this guy I'd only spoken to a few times. Just as I was about to suggest to Sarah that we go home and do something more productive with our Sunday, like paint our toenails, I saw Darren step out onto the top of the skateboard ramp. He was wearing a navy blue T-shirt that showed off his swallow tattoo and baggy Diesel jeans hung low on his hips so you could see the top of his Calvin Klein's. I decided I wasn't going anywhere. I couldn't take my eyes off him. As he soared down the ramp and leapt in the air, swinging his board around 360 degrees before landing, my stomach did somersaults with him. The sun was out, the crowds were cheering, the atmosphere was electric. And I was mesmerized.

"Pick your jaw up off the ground, Leyla. Show some dignity," Sarah said, bringing me back to reality with her sardonic tone.

"Wow!" was all I managed to say.

"You've lost it, you know. You've well and truly lost it. I've never seen you like this about anybody before."

"Shut up and let's get closer to the front. They're announcing the winner."

Sure enough, Darren won the championships and was paraded in front of the crowd on the tops of his friends' shoulders, brandishing a shiny trophy. I watched in awe before realizing that Darren was in fact waving at me. He gestured to his friends to let him down and walked over to me with a huge smile.

"We must stop bumping into each other like this. What are you doing here? I didn't think you were the skateboarding type, or is it another of your tricks, like being able to spin the discs?"

"Sarah wanted to come down for some reason. Her brother Jamie told her about it and she thought it would be cool, so she dragged me along. I was having a perfectly peaceful Sunday at home before she hauled me down here." I could feel my cheeks burning up and I imagined Sarah throwing back her head with laughter at the bullshit I was spouting.

"Well, I'm glad you came. Did you enjoy the show?"

"Yeah, it was cool. Where did you learn all that stuff?"

"Just knocking around the park for years watching the other kids. Mucking around, testing things out, you know." He looked around to see where all his mates were. People kept coming up and congratulating him. I didn't want to keep him from his moment of glory and started to go, but he stopped me and said that he just had to find Gary and Dean, and then wanted to know if I'd like to grab a Coke and go for a walk?

"I'll just have to find out what Sarah is up to," I said, trying to sound as cool as possible.

"I'll meet you at the amusement arcade in five minutes," he said, then staggered off into the crowd with his board and trophy.

Sarah was waiting for me with her arms folded, tapping her foot impatiently. "So you spoke to him. Are you feeling faint from the excitement? Do you need to sit down?"

"He's asked me to go for a walk with him, and you're coming too."

"No way. Uh-uh. You've got to be joking. I'm not playing gooseberry to anyone."

"You *have* to come. He'll be with his mates. He's just gone looking for them. Come on, Sarah, you're a total pro at these sorts of things. You can talk the hind legs off a donkey."

"Oh, thanks a bunch. So I'm supposed to entertain everyone on your behalf, am I?"

"No, I don't mean it like that. I mean you can break the ice. Abuse them about their goatees or pick a fight about Converse versus Nike trainers. Anything."

"Okay, okay. I'll come, but if he's not with his mates, I'm out of here. Right?"

"Okay, it's a deal."

We made our way over to the amusement arcade and found Darren with his two friends eating chips and taking turns on the Alpine ski simulator.

"Haven't you had enough of bombing down vertical slopes for one day?" Sarah asked Darren in a bored and unimpressed tone. I could tell she just thought he was showing off again.

"Funnily enough, I hate heights, but I think everyone should take the risk of falling at least twice a day. Don't you agree?" Darren smiled at her, waiting for a response.

I was expecting some immediate sarcastic quip from Sarah, but she stood contemplating him for a moment, trying to sum him up. You could see her turning her thoughts about him over and over in her head. I could tell she couldn't quite make him out, and an awkward silence grew. I was glad when Darren suggested we make a move. "Let's go for a walk. I'm sick of this place—it's full of kids."

We started off all walking alongside one another in a gang, talking about teachers and school, as that was the common ground between us all. I stayed close to Sarah and hid behind her jokes. Then Darren asked me if I still played the drums.

"Yeah, I still bash about. I've got my own kit at home, so I play around a bit. I'm not very good, but I do love playing them."

Sarah overheard me and interrupted. "She's brilliant.

Don't listen to a word she says about just bashing around now and again. She's too modest for her own good. Honestly, she spends hours practicing and has got a real talent for it. It's her life's passion."

Darren seemed genuinely interested, and pressed further. "Wow, that's amazing. It's so good to have something that you're really passionate about. You don't see many girls playing the drums, do you?"

"No, you don't, but there's no reason why they shouldn't. Girls just aren't encouraged to play them. I had to really fight to be allowed to play the drums at school. My mum and my music teacher were horrified. They thought I should be learning something more traditional and more becoming to a young girl, like the cello or the flute."

"So what made you want to play them in the first place?"

"I saw a band in concert on MTV one day and they had a girl drummer who was the coolest person I've ever seen and I decided there and then that I wanted to be just like her." Darren and I had fallen into step beside each other while the other three walked on ahead.

"I'd love to hear you," he said. "I play the guitar. Hey, we're practically a whole band. Out of everything I do, music is what I love the most. Skateboarding is just a bit of a hobby, you know? Just mucking around. But music is different."

"I don't do anything else except play the drums. My family thinks I'm a total weirdo. Sarah is very supportive and encouraging and everything, but I don't think she really understands or believes that I'm totally serious about making a career and a life out of it. All I want to do is be in a band and play the drums. Full stop. Nothing else. But most people find it difficult to imagine that dreams like that are possible, especially when you live round here where most girls are pregnant and engaged before they're twenty and a career at the bank is seen as a major achievement. I mean, each to their own and all, but I want more out of life than that. I don't want to be stuck in Bury for the rest of my days, getting old before my time, watching my dreams slowly fade away."

"It's easier said than done, though. You hear of so many people who all started out with these amazing dreams of becoming a footballer or traveling around the world or writing a book or whatever, and they all get to a stage where they've got to make a few decisions about their future and they suddenly become gripped by this fear and doubt. It's easier to just get a regular job, settle down with a nice girl, and work on a healthy bank balance. It's less effort and hassle, you know."

"I'm not just some naïve little kid with my head in the clouds—I do know that I've got a hell of a long way to go. It's going to take more hard work than I can imagine to achieve even a fraction of my dreams, but if I want it enough then it'll happen. I'm convinced of that."

"Well, good luck to you. I'm doing my guitar exams at the moment, and it's so much hard work that sometimes I just feel like jacking it all in and going down the pub with all my mates like any other normal eighteen-year-old."

"Where are you doing your exams?" I asked him.

"At the music college in Salford. I taught myself to begin with, but then I decided that I really wanted proper guitar lessons so that I could learn to read and write music and know exactly what I was doing when I was writing songs on my own."

"Apart from at school, I've only ever played on my own at home in the garage," I told him. "I've never really had an audience. I'm ready to start playing with other people now, though—there's only so much you can do on your own. Funnily enough, I've just had a really cool offer this weekend to get involved in some music workshops, teaching drums to a group of people who have never played an instrument before. We're probably going to write some music as well. I'm really excited about it."

Darren and I strolled through the park chatting comfortably about music, the bands we liked, the clubs we'd been to, the gigs we'd seen. My worries of not feeling confident or comfortable enough to talk to him were gone. Sarah was in the distance now, going as high as she could on the swings with Gary and Dean, and I didn't feel as though I needed her as my social crutch anymore.

"Look, there's the bandstand," Darren said, pointing at the crumbling domelike structure with the rusty ornate railings in the middle of the park. Many a brass band had entertained a parkful of summer picnickers from that bandstand. It hadn't been used for ages, though. An orange cordon was wrapped around the railings and a sign warned people to keep off the stage area because of subsidence.

"I'll race you there," I said, speeding off and getting a head start. Puffing and panting, I ducked under the cordon and ran onto the stage. It stank of urine, and there were empty condom and cigarette packets scattered about. Half-drunk bottles of strong cider stood at attention on benches that curved around the length of the semicircular stage. Darren eventually caught up with me and climbed inside the dome.

"Ugh, gross, it stinks in here," he said, turning up his nose.

"You'll play in worse places than this one day, when you're starting out, doing the pub circuit with your band," I joked, but I was half serious.

"No way. I'm going straight to the Albert Hall, darling."

Striking rock-star poses, jumping around playing air gui-tar, Darren and I pretended we were on stage at Wembley Stadium playing to a hundred-thousand-strong crowd. When we stopped to catch our breath, Darren put his hand on my shoulder and leant on me. His touch made goose bumps appear all over my forearms and down the back of my neck. Mucking around so much, I'd sort of forgotten how much I actually fancied him. But seeing him so close to me and feel-ing his touch made my heart beat faster. I stopped laughing and couldn't take my eyes off him. I didn't want him to ever move his hand from my shoulder. I don't know whether he sensed what I was feeling or whether he could read my mind, but he moved his arm farther along my back until it was around me and my head was resting against his shoulder. He squeezed gently, and slowly brought me round to face him. He was looking at me with a soft, warm smile. I didn't feel awkward or shy anymore. I didn't feel like I wanted to crawl out of his grip like I had done with so many boys before—the kind of boys who would just grab you, snog you, and go straight for your tits so that they could return to their mates bragging that they'd got to "second base." This felt different. I looked into his big green eyes and felt calm and happy. I put my face closer to his, and kissed him on the lips.

We held each other tightly and didn't speak. I didn't want to talk; any noise would have broken the moment. It's funny how you want those moments to last forever. But they always have to end. We heard Sarah and the others heading toward the bandstand, shouting our names.

"I really like you, Leyla," Darren whispered in my ear before the others interrupted us.

I looked him right in the eye and flashed him a big cheesy grin. What was the point in staring at the ground and being all coy about it? I felt great—he had made me feel great—and I didn't want to hide it. In fact, I wanted to run around the park and shout it to the whole world, but Sarah appeared and reminded us it was time to go home for our Sunday dinners.

EIGHT

ON WEDNESDAY NIGHT AFTER SCHOOL, I DECIDED TO go round to see Emma. I was still feeling really chuffed about Darren and couldn't help walking around with a grin on my face. I didn't fancy going straight home, where my good mood would be frowned upon and I'd be grilled with twenty suspicious questions.

Aunty Jean answered the door and waved me through to the living room, lighting up a fag on the way. A full ashtray spilled onto magazines and papers that were strewn over the coffee table next to a half-empty bottle of red wine and a dirty dinner plate. The ironing board was up in the corner of the room, with a basketful of washing waiting to be ironed by its side. Mum would have had a fit. Aunty Jean isn't dirty, but she isn't fussy about the state of her home like Mum is. Again I thought of how different they were; you'd never believe they were sisters.

Emma was on the phone in her bedroom. It was still a bit awkward between me and Aunty Jean. For just a short time when she opened the door everything would be normal and happy and easy, and then the reality of Emma's situation would descend once more. I often felt really guilty that I wasn't ill too. I felt as though I was a constant reminder to Aunty Jean of a girl practically the same age as Em, brought up almost identically, but with the one difference: that I didn't have HIV. I was always surprised that she didn't lash out more or ever feel the urge to grab me and tell me how unfair it all was. And it was unfair. Why Emma? I wondered whether Aunty Jean resented me and wished I wouldn't come round to remind her of the fact that I was healthy and her daughter wasn't.

We sat quietly on the sofa together. Aunty Jean flicked through a copy of *Hello!*, making the odd bitchy comment about some B-list celebrity draped over a chaise longue in a tasteless million-pound home. "These people might have money, you know, but they've got absolutely no style," she said, shaking her head in despair as she turned the page over to reveal the interior of yet another soap star's dreadful country cottage. On the telly Ricki Lake was encouraging some woman with big hair to tell the audience about how she'd found her husband in bed with her brother. I wished Emma would hurry up and get off the phone. I picked up a copy of *Cosmopolitan* from the coffee table and pretended to be engrossed so that Aunty Jean wouldn't feel the need to talk.

After a while I realized that she was being exceptionally quiet and had stopped making even the smallest remark. I looked up and noticed a few tears rolling down her cheeks. I strained my neck so as to see the article she was reading. From what I could gather it was about some actress whose daughter had cancer. She was fighting a daily battle with the disease and undergoing chemotherapy. The actress was telling the interviewer how touched and overwhelmed she'd been by the public's kindness and generosity. Her family had been inundated with cards, presents, donations, flowers, prayers, and advice.

Aunty Jean's face was drawn. I linked my arm through hers and squeezed tight. She pulled out a tissue that was tucked in her cardigan sleeve and mopped her eyes and blew her nose. "Oh, I'm sorry, Leyla. I shouldn't be crying in front of you like this."

"It's all right, I don't mind, honestly."

"It's just that, you know, when I read stories like that where there is so much public sympathy for a young girl who is tragically ill, I realize how different the situation is for families who are affected by HIV, whether they're rich or poor, famous or not. Imagine the response I'd get to my story about my sixteen-year-old daughter who had sex in the woods with some bloke she didn't know and contracted HIV. It just wouldn't be the same, would it?

"HIV is a dirty disease. That's what everyone thinks, anyway. I couldn't tell anyone that Em's got HIV. It's not socially acceptable to talk about it. It's best if it's kept our little secret. That's the worst thing about all of this, Leyla. I feel so alone. I know I've got to stay strong for Em, but there are times when I just want to break down and tell one of my friends and beg for help to get through all of this."

She cried into my shoulder. I suddenly felt really grown up. It felt odd and quite scary to have the roles reversed—me comforting good old Aunty Jean instead of the other way round for the first time in my life. God knows she'd mopped up enough of my tears over the years. I wanted to help, but I still felt panicky inside, like I wasn't sure how to handle it. At times, since Emma had told me about the HIV, I'd felt like a little girl who had been plonked in the middle of a totally grown-up situation with no guidebook, no rules or instructions on how to find my way around. I was scared of making a really big mistake, saying something stupid and making an already bad situation even worse. So I just kept quiet and held tightly on to Aunty Jean, hoping that my just being there would be enough.

Aunty Jean sat up suddenly and tossed the magazine onto the floor. "You won't be seeing any photos of me and Emma in some glossy magazine, sat together in our nice little flat, thanking the nation for its kindness. God, I could scream sometimes." She blew hard into her tissue.

Emma eventually came out of her room, looking pleased with herself. "You two look cozy. Any room for me?" she said, squeezing between us on the sofa.

"Who have you been talking to? You seem pretty chuffed," Aunty Jean probed, trying to act as normal as possible.

"I've been talking to Lucinda at the support center, and they're really excited about Leyla joining our music group. Leyla, they want you to come along this Saturday to meet everyone and find out about the plans for the music workshops," she said, turning to me with a slightly concerned look. "You haven't changed your mind, have you?"

Aunty Jean got up and offered to make us a drink.

"No, not at all. I've been practicing, actually. I didn't expect it to happen so quickly, though."

"They're just keen to get things moving. Quite a few people at the group are really excited about it all. They can't wait to get started."

"Oh God, I hope I can do it, Emma. I'm not sure I'm good enough yet to be teaching anybody."

"You'll be brilliant, and you won't be doing it single-handedly, anyway. There are going to be other musicians there."

"It feels strange to be called a musician. I only knock around on an old drum kit in my garage. I'm hardly a musician."

"You'd better start having more belief in yourself and stop being so modest, because you'll never make it big otherwise. You're a musician. Get used to it and start believing it." Emma gave me an encouraging smile. "I was thinking, though— what are you going to tell your parents you're doing every other Saturday?"

"Shit, I hadn't thought about that. How long will I be there for?"

"Well, it's eleven in the morning till five in the afternoon. I usually leave at about ten and get home at about six. Do you reckon they'll be really suspicious?"

"Yeah, probably, but I'm out practically every Saturday anyway doing something or other with you or Sarah."

"But you're going to have to leave at a regular time every week and literally be gone all day. You're almost never out of the house for the entire day. They'll begin to wonder what you're getting up to." Emma was starting to get a bit shrill. She jumped to her feet and seemed very agitated all of a sudden.

"I'll tell them that I've started drumming lessons in Manchester with a group of kids from our music class at school," I reassured her. "They'll buy that. They know I've wanted proper lessons for a while; I've just never got round to doing it. It's totally believable, and not that far from the truth, either, so I won't feel too bad about lying my arse off."

Emma had her back to me, and I could see her shoulders tense up. "This is awful. I hate all these lies. I've even got you lying to your parents now. I wish we could all be open and honest with one another. I just want to be normal. I hate all of these hushed, coded conversations and feeling like I've got to be looking over my shoulder wherever I go in case I'm doing something no one should know about. I hate it. Why don't I just tell everyone about the HIV and be done with it. I mean, what the hell are they all going to do to me anyway? Throw me in a pit and stone me to death or something?"

She was kicking newspapers and magazines about the floor. Her mood had changed dramatically, from being cheery and optimistic when she'd told me about the workshop to being at a boiling point with anger and frustration now.

"Listen, I'll just tell them that I'm going to a drum workshop. That's the truth, isn't it? I won't be lying at all then. It'll be fine. I don't have to tell them any more than that. I never tell them any details about my life anyway—they practically have to hold a gun to my head to get me to tell them what I want for my *tea*. It'll be fine," I said, trying to calm her down.

"That's not the point, Leyla."

I knew it wasn't the point, but I wanted to say something to make her feel better. I couldn't bear to just sit there yet again not knowing what to say or do.

"The point is that I'm sick of all these secrets and not being able to be honest about what's happening to me. It's driving me insane."

"Well, at least we'll go insane together, darling," Aunty Jean said in a calm, soothing tone. She was leaning against the living room door with her arms open to Emma. We hadn't even noticed that she was there; she must have heard everything. Emma went to her and fell into her arms. "I haven't got any answers for you, Em. I know all these secrets and lies are unfair and cruel, but it's just the way of the world. All I can think to do is blow the whole bloody planet up and start all over again. That's not very realistic, though, is it?" she said with a smile. But her attempt to diffuse Emma's anger wasn't successful.

Emma pulled herself away from Aunty Jean. "It shouldn't be this way, though. I can't be as complacent as you, Mum. I feel like I'm a walking time bomb about to go off any second. Why should I be made to feel so ashamed just because I've got this virus? I almost feel like society's cruelty could kill me before the HIV got a look in." Aunty Jean tried to put her arm around her, but Emma pushed her away. "Why has this happened to me? Why me? What the hell did I ever do wrong, eh?" she snarled, punching the living room door.

For one moment I really did think that she was going to lose it and trash the place or hurt someone—anyone, anything. I sat on the sofa with my knees drawn up to my chest and hugged myself, wanting to become as inconspicuous as possible. I couldn't stop thinking about Aunty Jean's outburst just a few minutes before Emma had come into the room. I didn't know how to handle the intensity of emotions. I felt completely out of my depth and wanted to disappear. It made me feel like a complete coward—a coward because I didn't have the guts to face their pain head-on. All I wanted to do was disappear out of there and go back to the happy thoughts of Darren and me that I'd walked into the flat with just half an hour earlier. I shut my eyes tight and buried my face in my arms for a couple of minutes, desperate to get my head together.

When I looked up, Emma was slowly beginning to unfurl herself from the tight knot she'd wound herself into. She relaxed her fists, unclenched her teeth, and flopped to the floor in a heap. Aunty Jean and I rushed to her and threw our arms around her. We all cried together, as much with relief at getting a lot of pent-up thoughts and feelings out in the open as anything else.

After we'd had some tea and calmed ourselves down, I quietly left the flat. Emma and I were so lucky to have her mum, I thought, because I didn't think I could handle it all on my own; the responsibility would just be too much. After the scene I'd just witnessed, I felt completely exhausted and emotionally drained. If I had to shoulder all of that on my own I think I would have collapsed under the pressure long before now. I wanted to help Em and Aunty Jean, but I was also aware that there was only so much I could do. I had to reassure myself that between me, her mum, her counselor, and the support group, Emma would be okay. I would be the best friend that I'd always been to Emma and help out in any way I could.

I was really late for tea and I knew Mum would be having a hairy fit, but our house is one big stifled emotion where absolutely no one talks about how they are feeling or what they really think about things, and the idea of going back there just wasn't appealing. Mum and Dad talk to each other about what needs doing in the house, what so-and-so did at work that day, or what they're having for tea. Sadie talks about Anthony and diets and gossips about her work colleagues. I couldn't remember a single time any of us had ever sat down with one another and had a heart-to-heart. It was probably as much my fault as anyone else's, but Mum and Dad never encouraged me to talk about my problems and refused to acknowledge that I had a personal life all of my own, so I never asked about theirs or about how life was treating them.

I suddenly felt a real urge to see Darren. I hadn't seen him since Sunday, and I knew he would do a good job of taking me out of myself, even if I couldn't talk to him about what had just gone on at Em's. My head was pounding with all the different images flashing through my mind. I could still see Emma bubbling over with anger and frustration, and Aunty Jean weeping into my shoulder, but I could also see Darren kissing me in the bandstand. Adrenaline soared through my veins, and I ducked into the next phone box I saw. I leafed through my address book, praying that I'd written Darren's number down from the scrap of paper he'd given me on Sunday. There it was, written in big bold letters under D.

I opened and closed the book a few times, making up my mind to call and then deciding against it. I was scared he'd think I was chasing him really hard and be totally put off. I was suddenly convinced that he didn't like me after all. But I'd been through all of this before, and every time I'd seen him he'd been really pleased to see me and had made me feel great about myself. I decided to take the plunge and just go for it.

I rang his number. Darren answered and sounded so surprised to hear from me that he almost dropped the phone. When I asked him if he fancied meeting me, instead of getting all flustered like I expected him to, he seemed genuinely excited and said that he'd meet me at the end of his road. I phoned Mum and told her I was going to Sarah's to finish off a history project that had to be in tomorrow.

I'd never felt this way about anyone before. I wanted to get to know this unbelievably cool guy so badly. I wanted him to like me. I had butterflies in my stomach and I kept checking myself in shop windows. I still had my school uniform on, so I didn't exactly look my best. I'd just have to dazzle him with my personality.

He was sat on a garden wall, and was staring down at his hands as I turned the corner. I saw him before he saw me, so I had a chance to gather myself and take a good look at him. He was as gorgeous as ever. He always looked so effortlessly cool. He glanced up and saw me, walked straight over, and kissed me hard on the lips.

"It's good to see you," he said.

"I was just on my way home from school, and was passing the music shop and thought of you. I knew you lived round here somewhere," I said, a little taken aback by the warm reception I was receiving.

"I was bored out of my brain doing English revision in my room. You rescued me. Listen, do you want to go back to mine or what? We could go down the chippy and sit out the back or I could show you my record collection if you're prepared to brave the weird and wonderful world of the Mitchell household."

The strain of what had just gone on at Em's and the stressful buildup to phoning Darren finally caught up with me, and I found myself shaking a little. I shivered and pulled my coat more tightly around me.

"You look freezing. Let's go back to mine. You'll have to excuse my parents, though. My mum will give you the third degree and try to work out who your family is and my dad will probably flirt with you, so we'll just say hi for two minutes and then make our excuses, okay? Just don't be too freaked out. They're all right really." He grabbed my schoolbag and carried it for me.

We started walking slowly back to his house. I wanted him to kiss me again. I couldn't quite believe the effect he had on me, to be honest. Being with him sent rushes of adrenaline through my body, and I had to stop myself from screaming with happiness. We got to the front door of his house and stepped into the glass porch, where shoes were lined up neatly next to a pottery umbrella stand in the shape of a duck. Their pebble-dashed semidetached house was identical to every other house on the road and beyond. A neat white picket fence bordered an immaculate lawn. There was a shiny beige BMW parked in the small gravel drive in front of the house. We hadn't even got in the hall properly when Darren's mum appeared. She was wearing a tracksuit and trainers and holding a glass of water.

"Oh, hello. You didn't tell me that we were expecting guests, Darren," she said, winking at me and flashing Darren a mischievous smile. She was very tall and slim and was wearing full makeup. She tapped the glass she was holding with long red manicured nails. Her hair was dyed an aubergine color and fell in bouncy curls around her shoulders. I imagined Mum summing her up in an instant: "Nouveau riche. Thinks she's better than everyone else. Her husband does a few dodgy deals, buys himself a flash car, and suddenly she thinks she's made it. Common as muck really."

"Uh, yeah, this is Leyla. She's a friend from school. She's a drummer. We're just going to listen to some music upstairs. Okay?" Darren tried to maneuver me in the direction of the stairs and away from his mum.

"Show your guest some hospitality, for goodness' sake, Darren. Would you like a drink, Leyla?"

"Um, yes please. A glass of orange would be great, thanks." I knew that wasn't the answer Darren wanted to hear, but I felt I had to be polite and not just rush on upstairs as soon as I'd walked in the door. I followed the aroma of expensive perfume into the kitchen.

"Come on through. You'll have to excuse the way I look. You've caught me in a right mess—I've just come back from my weekly aerobics class with the girls." She must have reapplied her makeup when she'd come out of the class, I thought, or else she couldn't have worked up any sweat whatsoever. She chattered away to me as she wandered around the fitted kitchen, fixing my drink and pulling different bits of food out of the fridge. She laughed at her own jokes and used her arms and hands a lot to express herself. I could see where Darren got part of his personality from. His mum was loud and extroverted and obviously liked being the center of attention.

Darren leant against the cooker, looking bored and agitated, desperate to get away.

"Our aerobics instructor was telling us tonight about a couple of young girls, probably no older than you, Leyla, who had come into her class a few weeks back full of energy, raring to go. They really went for it: running around the room at top speed, doing sit-ups at a hundred miles an hour, practically bouncing off the walls. They were in the shower room afterward when one of them collapsed and had to be taken away in an ambulance. It turns out they'd both taken amphetamines before they'd come to the class—just to see what it would be like. It backfired, of course. It's terrible what young kids do these days for a bit of entertainment. They're ruining their lives."

Darren and I looked at each other and just burst out laughing. The idea of these two girls getting off their heads on speed and then doing a full hour of aerobics in first gear was just too funny.

Darren's Mum wasn't very amused that we found her story so hilarious and frowned at us both sternly. I went bright red and wished I could disappear. Sensing my embarrassment, Darren tried to make it up with his mum and gave her a hug to lighten the atmosphere. She seemed to appreciate his gesture and carried on chatting.

"How's about a bite to eat?" she asked. "I've got pizza slices, chicken nuggets—oh, and I might have a couple of spring rolls I could throw in the microwave."

"Mum is the queen of finger food. Her idea of a hearty Sunday dinner is a tube of Pringles and a selection of dips from Marks & Spencer." Darren kissed her on the cheek to let her know he was only teasing. "My dad's definitely the cook in this house."

"Well, that's what all that women's lib stuff was about, wasn't it? Telling us women to get out of the kitchen. I can't be bothered fussing with food anyway. I'd rather let Terry get on with it so that I have more time to make myself look beautiful." She ran her fingers through her curls and giggled.

"Listen, Mum, we just want to go and listen to some records. Leyla will have to go home soon," Darren said gently.

"Yeah, thanks for the drink," I said, and followed Darren out of the kitchen.

As Darren closed his bedroom door behind him, he breathed a huge sigh of relief. "Thank God my dad didn't spot you—we'd *never* have got away. She's a bit full-on, isn't she? Sorry about all that drugs stuff—she's got a real thing about them. She's terrified that I'm going to turn into some sort of druggy 'cos I'm out DJing in clubs all the time. She reads all that stuff in the newspapers about E and is totally convinced that I'm going to die from popping a pill one night. She was just sussing out your reaction to the speed story, I reckon. Trying to work out if you're some sort of junkie that I've picked up at a club."

"I shouldn't have laughed, should I?"

"No way—she's a total hypocrite. She's reaching for her Prozac every five minutes. I learnt to say 'Valium' before I could say 'Mummy' or 'Daddy' when I was little."

"You seem very close to her, though. She's very glamorous for a mum."

"She's bricking it about getting old and losing her looks. She spends hours on her makeup and going to the gym and all that stuff. My dad had an affair with a twenty-one-year-old woman about five years ago and they nearly got divorced over it, but my mum decided to take him back. So now she's completely paranoid about her looks and is convinced that Dad's going to dump her for a younger model when she's past it. It's really sad, when you think about it. She'll probably end up being one of those hideous plastic women who has had so much surgery done to her face that she'll barely be able to talk."

"God, how did you cope with your dad having that affair?"

"I just hid away from it all in my bedroom and buried myself in music. That's when I started to learn to play the guitar. I used to spend hours up here practicing chord changes to drown out the rows that were going on downstairs. I suppose it made me and Mum quite close, though. I sort of looked after her." Darren had absentmindedly picked up his acoustic guitar and was strumming out a few chords. "Anyway, that's all depressing shit. We're young and free and won't be making the same mistakes as those idiots, so who cares?"

Darren walked over to his Technics decks and put a record on. I was stood in the middle of the room taking in his books and his posters and especially his records when he took me by the hand and pulled me down to lie next to him on the bed. My heart was pounding by now, and I was convinced it was so loud that Darren must be able to hear it. I couldn't actually believe that I was lying with Darren on his bed. He ran his hand down my back and rested it on my thigh. He pulled me closer to him so that our faces were inches apart, and we sank into each other's eyes. I trembled with excitement as he brought his hand up to touch my face, and brushed against my breast as he did so. He gently stroked my cheek and kissed me, first on each of my eyelids and then on my lips. I was in heaven.

How on earth had this all happened? Two and a half weeks ago we'd bumped into each other at a gig and next thing, we were tickling each other's tonsils in his bedroom. It seemed to have happened so fast, and so naturally. I hadn't stopped thinking about him and fancying him from afar ever since we'd met at the gig, and he'd made every effort with me whenever we'd seen each other, so it just felt right. It felt fantastic, in fact.

"So are we . . . you know, seeing each other properly like, or what?" Darren asked, propping himself up on his elbow after we'd kissed in silence for ages.

I was shocked at how direct he was. There was no messing about or playing any games. I was used to all the crap you usually have to go through with boys: pretending that you don't really fancy them, having a snog and then acting like it never happened, never saying what you're really thinking, pretending not to care when you see them with their hand up someone else's skirt.

There was none of that with Darren, so far at least. He was being totally straight with me. And I wasn't complaining. This was obviously the advantage of falling for an older guy. I stumbled over my answer to his question. "I, urm, guess so if that's what you want. I mean, it's what I want too, it's just . . . God, this feels weird, but then it doesn't, either, it feels completely normal, but weird as well. Oh no, stop me, I'm rambling." I covered my face with my hands and fell back on the bed.

"Listen, I really like you a lot. You've got a total mind of your own, like you're making up your own rules as you go along. You're really sorted. All the girls I've ever been out with before have just been bothered about their weight, their hair, and who's snogging who at school. It's boring, you know, and you're the opposite of all that." He leant over to kiss me, and it felt brilliant.

"So is that it? Are we, like, 'an item'?" I asked.

"Yes, you are now mine. You are forever in my power." Darren reached over to the amp at the side of his bed and picked up a thin plain silver bracelet. He slid it onto my wrist. "You will wear the slave bangle and remain in my control."

I twisted it around on my wrist, admiring it. "God, it's lovely. Where did you get it?"

"I found it when I was DJing one night. Keep it, it suits you."

I glanced at my watch and noticed how late it was getting. Mum would be phoning Sarah's to find out where I was if I didn't get home soon. "I'd better get going, Darren. I don't want to walk home too late," I said, and eased myself reluctantly off the bed.

"I'll walk you home. It's too dark for you to go walking around here on your own."

As we walked and talked, I kept sneaking glances at the bracelet he'd given me. I was overwhelmed by my feelings toward him. I was practically seeing stars. It was all I could do to stop myself from jumping up and down with excitement. I was going out with the fittest bloke in school. I could hardly believe it.

"Have you started going to that music workshop you told me about yet?" Darren asked, snapping me out of my reverie.

I'd completely forgotten that I'd told him about the workshop, and it made me think about Em again. I hoped she was all right and wasn't feeling too freaked out by the emotional scene that had taken place at the flat. "No, not yet, but I'm going next Saturday actually. Any tips?"

"Always look like you know what you're doing. Winging it is half the challenge."

When I got home I sneaked up the stairs and called from the landing to let them know I was back. I ran into my room and flopped down on my bed, twisting my brand-new bracelet round and round my wrist. I let out a small yelp of delight.

"Are you all right in there?" Mum shouted from her bedroom.

Our stupid paper walls—you could hear everything. I was annoyed that Mum had invaded my private thoughts, but I couldn't take the grin off my face. "I'm fine," I shouted back curtly. I'm fine, I thought. I'm fantastic.

NINE

ON THE SATURDAY OF MY FIRST TRIP TO THE SUPPORT center with Emma, I went downstairs to have breakfast with Mum and Dad before making my way down to Em's, where a taxi would pick us up. I'd told them that I was going to a music workshop in town with a group of people from my music class at school and that it would be something I'd be doing every fortnight for a while.

They couldn't quite get it into their heads that I might want to do something slightly more interesting with my Saturdays than hang around the makeup section of Boots with the other girls my age or sit drinking endless cups of tea with Mum and Sadie in the upstairs café of British Home Stores. That's what Saturdays are for round here. The men go to the football, the women go shopping, the kids play on the street, then they all get together at the end of the day to fall asleep in front of the telly. The idea that anyone could possibly think about doing anything different blows their minds.

"So where are you going again?" Dad asked, folding his paper away as Mum presented him with the usual fry-up. I took a deep breath and as calmly as possible told him my plans for the third time. "I'm going to a music workshop to practice my drums and to learn how to work with other musicians."

"And what do you get at the end of it, a certificate or something?"

"You don't get anything at the end of it. It's just a chance for me to practice with other people instead of drumming on my own in the garage all the time."

"At least you won't be making a racket round here and be ruining the street's peace and quiet," Mum chipped in.

Dad still wasn't satisfied with what I'd had to say. "So you won't even get a qualification out of it. Seems a bloody waste of time to me. You want to start thinking about a career, my girl. You should be out getting yourself a nice Saturday job: learning some skills, making yourself useful, earning some money. Not faffing around on those drums. Have you not got any idea what you want to do later in life?"

He looked up from his plate and frowned at me, demanding some sort of explanation. I noticed that he had egg yolk dripping down his chin. Ever since I was little, money is all Dad has ever thought about. I stood looking at him eat his breakfast and remembered the time we went to the dogs together one Friday night after school when I was about twelve. Dad's dog came in first and we drove home throwing bundles of five-pound notes into the air. It took me until we got back to the house to count it all. That was probably the last time me and Dad had done anything together properly.

"How many times have I got to tell you? I want to be a drummer." I was beginning to lose my patience. It infuriated me the way they didn't take me seriously, treating me like some stupid kid.

"That's not a proper career, that's a hobby. How are you going to earn a living, bring up a family, afford a mortgage? The sooner you wake up to the real world and start learning some useful skills for the job market the better, young lady."

It was the patronizing "young lady" tacked on the end that nearly sent me over the edge, but I caught myself before there was a scene that would no doubt lead to me being banned from leaving the house altogether. "Music is a serious business, Dad, and plenty of people spend their lives devoted to it. Just because I'm not reaching for the dizzy heights of becoming regional manager of Abbey National, as Sadie so obviously is, doesn't mean I don't have ambitions or a career plan," I said in the calmest voice I could muster. "Oh, and by the way, you've got egg on your face."

"Me and Sadie are going to the factory shop this afternoon," Mum chipped in. "You can get all the designer gear for half the price, you know. I got your dad some Levi's the other week. Dirt cheap they were. Why don't you come with us, Leyla. You can go to this workshop thing another time. Come on. We'll get chips on the way home for tea."

I felt a bit sorry for Mum. She was trying, I suppose. She just didn't understand what I was doing. Me and Mum don't get on half the time and we might as well be from different planets, but I do still love her. "Mum, I can't. This workshop is really important to me. Look, I'm late as it is. I'd better go. Save me some chips for tea if you get some." I picked up my toast and ran out of the door.

Walking along the high street toward Emma's flat, I couldn't help but wonder how my parents would react if they knew the real reason for these workshops. They'd go spare for so many different reasons that I didn't even want to think about. All I knew was that I was doing the right thing and no matter how much trouble I could get into I was prepared for it, because I had to help Emma somehow.

Emma was waiting for me when I arrived. I hadn't seen her since Wednesday, when we'd all got really upset, but I was glad to see that she was in much better form. I was feeling pretty nervous, as I wasn't sure what to expect at the workshop and whether I would be able to handle what I was going to experience. And I wasn't really sure what was expected of me. I knew that I would be spending the day with a group of people around my age who knew of their own or a family member's HIV status. But I wasn't sure if I was meant to be a counselor or something like that. I was terrified of saying the wrong thing. I still didn't know enough about HIV, and there was a lot of stuff that scared me stupid about it.

I must have been quieter than usual thinking about all of these issues, because Emma was suddenly hugging me and telling me how lucky she was to have a friend like me.

The taxi arrived and took us into town. It was a half-hour ride, giving Emma and me plenty of time to catch up on each other's news.

"So have you seen that Darren lad again, the one who was DJing at that party we went to?"

"Well, actually there have been one or two developments since I last saw you," I said, keeping her in suspense but dying to tell her all about it at the same time. "He asked me out, actually."

Emma gasped and punched me in the leg. "I don't believe it. How did that happen without me knowing about it. Come on, spit it out."

"Me and Sarah went down to this skateboard tournament last weekend at the park with her brother Jamie. It turns out that Darren was competing in it. Anyway, I met up with him afterward and we all went for this big walk together. Me and Darren seemed to break off from the rest of the gang and ended up messing around in the bandstand, pretending we were rock gods playing to an audience of thousands. It was hilarious. He's such a good laugh."

"Then what? Come on, you're killing me."

"Well, then we ended up kissing before we went home."

"In that stinky old bandstand?"

"Yeah, well, I wasn't really bothered about my surroundings to be honest, Em," I said sarcastically.

"But one kiss doesn't necessarily mean you're going out with him. Something else must have happened."

"Hold your horses. I went round to his house on Wednesday after I saw you and we went out on Friday night. Well, we didn't exactly go out—we nicked a bottle of his dad's red wine and sat in the park by his house." I giggled nervously as a wave of excitement came over me in thinking about him and the fact that I was actually seeing him properly.

Emma let out a little scream and kissed me on the cheek. "I bet Sarah is pleased. Not!"

"I think she might have come round to liking him, actually. She knows that I'd never go out with a complete loser. She's got to trust me when I say that he's the most gorgeous, funny, intelligent, sensitive, talented guy on earth and he luurves me. He gave me this bracelet."

Emma oohed and aahed over the bracelet and told me how happy she was for me. It can't have been easy for her. Talking about boys in that way was bound to remind her of her one-night fling that ended in disaster in Wales. But she seemed to take my news in her stride.

We eventually arrived at the center. My nerves came back as we walked through the doors, but I was soon made really welcome by Lucinda and Graham, another of the center's coordinators. They had already heard all about me. The center was made up of one light and airy hall with wooden floorboards and big, comfy sofas and several other smaller meeting rooms that led off from the hall. A lot of people had already arrived and were chatting in different groups in the main area. I had expected to see really ill people in wheelchairs with no hair and gaunt faces, but everyone there looked like anyone else out on the street. We could have been in any café in town.

I found myself breathing a sigh of relief. I could only cope with one thing at a time. Emma still looked and acted so normal, and although there were a few changes, like the food and tablets I knew she had to take, her life went on pretty much as usual. I hadn't really thought too much about the fact that she could get seriously ill. I knew I had a long way to go in truly coming to terms with Emma's illness. So far I had only begun to think about all of the outside prejudice and having to hide Emma's status from our family and friends. I knew that I had plenty more hurdles to get over.

Lucinda and Graham asked if they could have a private word with me to talk through a few things about the center while Emma went off to join the teenage group. They said they knew that I was the only other person apart from her mother in Emma's immediate circle of family and friends who knew of her status, and they recognized that I must be coming to terms with a lot of stuff myself. It was as though they'd read my mind.

They hoped that being a part of the group would be good for me, as it was an environment where issues around HIV were discussed and problems shared. And they felt that it would be excellent for Emma to have someone in her family who was learning as much about living with HIV as she was, so that she wouldn't feel entirely alone and isolated when she was away from the center. They explained that in no way was I at the center to act as a counselor or supervisor and that I could drop any role of responsibility that I might have assumed around Emma. My role in the workshop was purely to teach drumming and to help put some music together.

They also talked to me about confidentiality, about how vitally important it was to the safety and well-being of all those attending the center that everyone I saw there and everything I heard there never left the premises. I was certainly feeling more relaxed by the time they showed me the way to the room where Emma's group was and invited me to start taking the drumming lessons on the following Saturday at the music college.

I spotted Emma sat on one of the sofas over by the drinks machine. She was talking to a girl with long dark hair, olive skin, and big pouting red lips. There were about twenty people in the room, including three staff. Some of the girls were reading magazines, a few people were getting rowdy as they competed with one another at a PlayStation in the corner of the room, and others were just stood around chatting or choosing CDs to put on the stereo. It was a perfectly relaxed atmosphere, and nobody batted an eyelid when I walked in the door.

I went over to the drinks machine to get myself a Coke, not wanting to interrupt Emma but at the same time hoping that she'd see me.

"Leyla, there you are. Come and sit down here with us." She turned to the girl sat next to her and quietly asked her if she minded me joining them.

I didn't want to intrude on them and sit there like a spare part. "It's all right, I'm fine over here. There's a magazine I want to read anyway."

"Don't be daft. Get your arse over here now," the girl said, on her feet and making space for me on the sofa.

I grabbed my Coke and walked over to them. Emma spoke quietly and nervously and kept her eyes low. I hadn't ever seen her look so tense around other people before. It threw me, because I was supposed to be the uptight one. "This is Ellie. Ellie, this is my cousin Leyla."

"Good to meet you," Ellie said. "You must be the drummer. I can't wait for the music group to start, though I don't think I'm coordinated enough for the drums. I'll stick to playing the triangle, I reckon."

Ellie had turned slightly toward me and had her back to Emma, but I could see over her shoulder that Emma's eyes had glazed over and she was staring blankly into space. I wondered what they had been talking about before I'd arrived and wished I hadn't interrupted them. I was struggling to make conversation with Ellie and tried to remember what Emma had told me about her.

"Emma told me you were a singer," I said eventually.

"Not exactly. My mum used to sing. She played all the clubs in Toronto when I was little, before she died. She used to prop me up in the dressing rooms of these smoky bars

while she did her turn. So I've always wanted to sing and follow in her footsteps." She put on a false razzle-dazzle smile
and in a high-pitched American accent sang, "There's no
bizzness like show bizzness."

She was cool. I liked her immediately. But I wished Emma
would join in and snap out of her trance. She'd usually have
been doing high kicks and cartwheels to accompany Ellie's
sparkling performance.

"So when's the workshop starting?" Ellie asked me.

"Next week, apparently. I think they're going to talk about
it with everyone today and decide who wants to do what." I
leant over and touched Emma's knee to get her attention.
"What are you going to do, Em?"

She was miles away. "What? Do what? What are you talking about?"

"The music workshop. What are you going to do?"

"Oh, I dunno. Sing I suppose."

"Emma and her mum do karaoke down the Butcher's
Arms practically every Friday night. She's got a great voice," I
said encouragingly, hoping to engage Emma. But she just sank
back farther into the sofa and stared at her hands. "Listen, I'll
leave you two to it. Sorry I interrupted you." I started to get
up, but Ellie told me to sit down and turned to Emma to give
her a quick hug.

"Don't go. I was only telling Emma about my boyfriend
troubles. Are you going out with anyone?"

It was obvious that that was why Emma was upset. It had
probably sparked off all sorts of thoughts about boyfriends
and sex. I didn't want to go into my new relationship with
Darren and make things even worse. I'd gone on about him
enough in the taxi. I shrugged my shoulders and avoided eye

contact with Ellie, hoping that she'd change the subject.

"Come on, don't be coy. Tell Ellie about the DJ you're seeing who you're going to live happily ever after with in pop heaven." Emma let a timid smile creep across her face but stayed slumped in the back of the sofa.

"I knew I shouldn't have told you," I said teasingly. "His name's Darren. He's in the upper sixth at my school and he's just, I dunno, really nice. We've only just started going out."

"And he's the funniest, most gorgeous, intelligent, sensitive guy on earth," Emma added.

I rolled my eyes and turned to Ellie to ask why she was having problems with her boyfriend, eager to take the spotlight off me.

"Oh God, it's really complicated." Ellie drew in her breath and rubbed her forehead as though she'd got a headache just thinking about it. Emma stayed where she was, biting her nails and acting like she wasn't really listening. "I've been seeing this guy David for about five months now. He's a friend of a friend. There's a gang of us who always hang around with each other 'cos we all left school at the same time when we were sixteen and we've stuck together. I met him when we were all out at a club one night. He's really cool, you know, and we get on like a house on fire. The only thing is, he doesn't know about me being, you know . . . HIV positive. I mean, he knows something's wrong because he's seen my hospital appointment cards in my room, but I've told him it's to do with my asthma. It's hard hiding it from him, but I've never had the confidence to tell him. It's not that I don't trust him—I'm just scared of rejection. I really like him and don't want to lose him, I guess." Ellie played with her long dark hair and looked across the room, not meeting Emma's or my eyes. I noticed tears spring to her eyes. Emma slowly and cautiously reacted and gently put her hand over Ellie's.

"So anyway, it's got to the stage now that David wants to have sex with me," Ellie continued. "He's my first serious boyfriend really, and I've never had sex with anyone before, but if there's anyone I want to do it with, it's David. We're both seventeen, we've been going out for quite a while, and we really love each other, so David doesn't understand what the problem is. I'm amazed he's been so patient; not many lads would wait so long to get their leg over. Every time we've got close to, you know, making luurve, I've just brought things to a grinding halt, sharpish-like. David has been pretty understanding so far, saying that he doesn't want to push me into doing anything I don't want to do, but there's going to come a time soon when he'll lose patience and want a good explanation from me." Ellie sighed and slouched back, looking deflated.

"It's not as if I don't want to have sex with him, because I do. He's gorgeous, for God's sake. I'm *gagging* to rip his clothes off. But even if we take precautions and I convince him to wear double condoms or something so that there's as little risk as possible, I still feel that I should tell him my status before we have sex. It's only fair to him, so that he can make a proper decision after he's heard all the facts. I'm just too scared to tell him. I don't want him to run a mile—I like him too much."

I was gobsmacked. There's no other way to describe how I felt listening to this seventeen-year-old girl telling us that she couldn't have sex with her boyfriend because she was too frightened to tell him she was HIV positive. The world should have been her oyster. She was young, crowd-stoppingly beautiful, totally clued up—she should have had the world kneeling at her feet. Instead, she couldn't just enjoy an exciting new relationship with her horny boyfriend, because not only did she have to think about the usual worries of having sex for the first time, but she also had her status to consider.

But the fact that she was a virgin and HIV positive puzzled me. I wondered how she'd got it in the first place.

Emma was amazing. She sat up straight and just listened and didn't try to tell Ellie what she should do. She didn't interrupt and start talking about her own experiences. She just made it easy for Ellie to open up and talk. No one came to any conclusions or came up with any groundbreaking solutions. It must have felt good for Ellie just to be able to talk about it.

"I've just got to go away and ask myself a few more questions," Ellie was saying. "I've decided that I'm always going to tell a partner about the HIV before I have sex with them. I've just got to work on this awful fear of rejection. I want to live as normal a life as possible, and to do that I'm going to have to work out a way of telling people whom I love and trust about my status, in the hope that they'll be able to help me live an ordinary life. Hmm, there's so much to think about." She closed her eyes and drifted off into her own space. Emma and I sat quietly on either side of her, thinking about what she'd just told us. There were issues that hadn't even entered my mind.

I felt helpless and naïve again, and wondered how Emma was feeling; I wished there were some magic words to say. Lucinda came in and broke our silence. She asked if we could all gather together to talk about a few things. I had to introduce myself, which I was a bit embarrassed about. Whenever I'm in those situations with a whole bunch of people whose eyes are all turned on me, my mind goes blank and I almost forget my own name. I'm always surprised when a little voice croaks out the right information.

Once the introductions were over and done with, we moved on to heavier issues and were told that Shula, who was sat in the circle opposite me, was having a lot of problems at home. Lucinda explained that Shula had allowed her to bring Shula's situation up in the group. She told us that Shula's family members were experiencing severe harassment from their neighbors, who had somehow found out that Shula's mum was HIV positive. With the sole aim of forcing the family out of the neighborhood, these neighbors were executing a reign of terror against her and her family. They had sprayed the wall of Shula's house with graffiti, spat on family members as they left the house, and taunted Shula as she walked to school. As a result, Shula's mum had decided to move away from the area and start a new life.

Lucinda just told us the bare facts of the situation and nothing else. She said that she wanted to bring the issue of harassment to the group and hear people's thoughts, personal experiences, fears, worries. Rafi, an Asian boy wearing a red baseball cap backward, was sat to the right of me. He volunteered to speak first. He told us about the racial harassment he often encountered at school, where white kids would tell him to go home to Pakistan and get out of their country. He told us that he'd never even stepped foot in Pakistan and that he had lived in Rusholme all his life. He had a thick Manchester accent and seemd exactly like any other lad in Manchester. His skin color was the only difference.

I could feel myself begin to panic about what I was going to say. I was terrified of saying something stupid or totally inappropriate. Some people had spoken, some hadn't. Lucinda asked if I wanted to say anything, and although it would have been easy to say nothing and let them move on to the next person, I found myself talking about the incident on the netball court a few weeks previously, when Claire Higgins had been bullying Teresa Glass. I told the group how popular, confident, and beautiful Claire Higgins was always picking on Teresa Glass because she was a bit of a loner and had a gum disease that was causing her teeth to rot. I described how Claire had taunted Teresa about her teeth and had encouraged her friends to join in and had then deliberately tripped Teresa up on the court so that she fell and cut her chin open. I went on to explain how horrified and angry I'd felt, but that I had walked away complaining of stomach cramps so I could be excused from the games lesson.

"I felt so ashamed later for not sticking up for Teresa. I'd just backed away instead of confronting Claire. It still makes me feel bad thinking about it now. I've always thought that if I was being bullied someone was bound to come to my rescue, but if I'm any example to go by I'd be left for dog meat." I looked down at my hands instead of facing the group members, who were all silently listening to my story. Lucinda thanked me for sharing my experience with the group, and asked if anyone else had anything to say.

After the discussions were brought to a close, the pizzas they'd ordered for lunch arrived and everyone fell into their own small groups again. Shula came over with a liter bottle of lemonade and a pizza to sit with Ellie and Emma on the sofa.

"Those girls on the netball court sound like right idiots," Ellie said. "If I was you, though, I'd have told everyone that I'd marched on in there on a crusade to eradicate bullying from schools once and for all. Made myself into a bit of a superhero. Then again, you only admitted to doing what everyone in this room would probably have done." Ellie smiled at me and passed a plateful of veggie pizza over.

"I thought I'd completely forgotten about it actually, but it's obviously been in the back of my mind since it happened," I told her.

Shula moved to the edge of the sofa and, finishing off a mouthful of pizza, said timidly, "It made me think of all the people who walk on past when our nightmare neighbors from hell are laying into one of us. I've always cursed the people who just shuffle on by, heads down, wishing they were invisible, but maybe it's stayed with them for a long time afterward like it has with you, and they might act differently next time."

"I reckon I'd butt in next time for sure," I said, nodding vigorously.

"So where are you moving to? Do you know yet?" Emma asked.

"Mum wants to move away from Manchester completely. She wants a fresh start where no one knows us. She's thinking of Leeds or Sheffield, but who knows, we might end up staying put with any luck." Shula tutted and didn't seem very impressed by her mum's idea.

"So you're not too keen on moving away, then?" Emma asked sympathetically.

"I'm just knackered. Mum's been really ill recently and her eyesight is going, so she depends on me even more than usual now. I have to do most of the housework when I get home from school, and I do all the cooking. I mean, I want to help Mum, but sometimes it just gets a bit too much. And all of this hassle from our neighbors is doing my head in. Mum barely leaves the house because she's so terrified of them, and she just cries all the time."

"You've got to get out of there. I'd be out of there in a flash," Ellie chipped in, shaking her head in disbelief over the situation.

"Yeah, but I can't help thinking that we're only going to get the same hassle somewhere else. Someone will find out about my mum eventually and the same thing will happen all over again. I don't think I could handle another move. Mum doesn't realize how hard it is to settle in at a new school. It's just doing my nut in."

We carried on talking for ages, until someone came round with a sheet of paper and asked us to write down what we each wanted to do the following Saturday at the workshop. At that point the conversation turned to music, and stayed on it.

Emma and I were pretty subdued in the taxi on the way home. My mind was full of all the new people I'd met and all their different stories of how HIV affected their lives. It had been a full-on day, but I was glad I'd gone along. It had opened my eyes up anyway.

"What did you think to the place then?" Emma eventually asked when we were about halfway home. We had to keep our voices down so that the taxi driver didn't hear us and find anything out about the center he'd just picked us up from. We huddled closer together on the backseat.

"I'm glad I went. I reckon it'll be really good for you, Em, being able to talk about all the different problems and everything."

"It wasn't too heavy? I was worried at one point that it was getting a bit too intense, with some of the stories people were coming out with."

"Nah, I can handle it. I'm hard, me," I reassured her. "I was worried about you, though. You were so quiet when I first came into the room. Had you been talking to Ellie about boyfriends?"

"Hmm, yeah. Sorry about that. I didn't exactly help you to fit in, did I? It just got me thinking about whether I'm ever going to have another boyfriend, and how I'd cope with it even if I did. You heard Ellie worrying about having sex with her bloke and telling him about her status, and that's with someone she loves and trusts. I should be playing the field a bit at my age, enjoying meeting different people and going out with different lads. I'd be too frightened to have sex with anyone again now; I'd be scared of giving it to them. So it doesn't look as though I'll ever have a normal relationship with anyone ever again." Emma moved away from me and thumped her head against the car window so hard the taxi driver turned round to see what had made the noise.

"Watch it, Em, you'll hurt yourself. Come on, of course you'll have more relationships. You might just have to wait for the right guy to come along, someone who is mature and understanding enough to deal with the situation, that's all. There are people like that out there, you know. Besides, that's what the center's there for. I'm sure they'll be able to help you sort things like that out in your head. You're lucky you've got that place, Em. What do other kids like you do if there isn't a support group like Positive Living near them? Are there places like it all over the country?"

"I don't think so. There aren't many places at all for teenagers with HIV. There must be somewhere in London, but I don't reckon they're all over the place. Some of the people at Positive Living have to travel miles to get there."

"God, imagine if you were living in the middle of the countryside in Scotland or something and you had no one to turn to."

"Well, if Mark in *EastEnders* is anything to go by, you wouldn't need a support center or any counseling whatsoever. You'd have your entire neighborhood rallying around for you and you wouldn't ever have to go to hospital for checkups or take a bucketload of tablets every five seconds without anyone knowing about it, so you'd probably be just fine." Emma shuffled around in her seat and eventually put her head down on my lap. "Wake me up when we get home. I could sleep for a hundred years."

"Em, just one thing before you go to sleep. It's been bugging me. How did Ellie get ill if she hasn't ever had sex?"

"She's had it since she was born. She got it from her mum. Her mum died of AIDS a while ago." Emma was tired and groggy. "I just want to sleep, Leyla."

The taxi crawled through the heavy Saturday afternoon traffic. Everyone was pouring out of the match and football lads celebrating a win banged on the roof of the car, singing and chanting. Dad would be coming out soon as well, and I had images of him spotting me in the taxi and seeing Emma. More excuses. I stroked Em's hair protectively. The secret was beginning to get bigger and bigger.

TEN

THE SATURDAY OF THE FIRST MUSIC WORKSHOP
arrived sooner than I expected. The week at school seemed to
fly by, and before I knew it my alarm was going off on
Saturday morning, telling me to get up and get drumming. I
wanted to have a quick warm-up session in the garage before
I left, so I jumped in the shower and got ready in record time.
I was on a roll, really concentrating on getting a drum
sequence right to a particularly difficult tune, when Mum
burst in and yanked my headphones off.

"Oi! I was in the middle of practicing. I've got to go to my
workshop in a minute," I said, scowling.

"It's your sister's birthday on Monday. It's her twenty-
first."

"Yeah, I know. She's been broadcasting it to the nation for
weeks."

"I thought it would be a nice idea for us all to have a special family day out together to celebrate. She's having a bit of a do with Anthony and her mates down at the Bull and Gate on Monday night, so I thought we could celebrate as a family today."

"Today?" I screeched incredulously.

"Yes, today. Your dad suggested we get in the car and drive to Bakewell or Matlock and enjoy a bit of the countryside, get out of the city."

"Mum, you know I have my drumming lessons on Saturdays. This is only my second week. I can't miss one so soon."

"Leyla, it's your sister's twenty-first. What's more important, them drums or your own flesh and blood?"

"Mum, don't be so ridiculous. You're not exactly giving me much notice, are you? You can't just come in here five minutes before I'm about to leave and expect me to change all my plans."

"Well, excuse me, madam. I didn't realize we had to book an appointment in your diary these days."

Dad, still in his dressing gown and hardly looking as though he was all geared up for a day out in the country, heard our raised voices from the kitchen and came in to see what all the fuss was about. "What's going on? Are you two at it again?"

"Madam over there seems to think that bashing around on some instrument all day is more important than her family and won't come out with us to celebrate Sadie's twenty-first," Mum said calmly but firmly.

"I only suggested that it might be a good idea to have a quick spin, seeing as it's a nice day, love," Dad said to Mum, a quizzical look on his face, obviously amused as to why it had all become such a big deal.

"Oh, and Mum turns the idea of a 'quick spin' into a big family affair and then plays on my guilty conscience so that I'll be forced to come with you," I retorted.

"Nobody's forcing you to do anything, love, but your mother's right: You don't spend enough time with us, and maybe we should have more family outings."

"Well, if you could just give me a little more notice next time maybe there won't be such a scene. But why you have to make me feel so bad for going to these workshops, I don't know. Is it going to be like this every time, because if it is you're wasting your breath. I'm going, and that's final."

I was sick of storming out on my parents all the time, but they drove me mad. The irony was that I was in fact bending over backward to be with a member of my family who was in dire need of my love and support. If only they knew. And if only Mum had a better relationship with her own sister we could all be a lot more open with one another; I wouldn't have to be hiding this big family secret from them, and they might understand me better.

At the center, I met up with the three other people who had been asked to take the workshop. One of them, Glen, is Lucinda's brother. He plays the guitar, so she managed to convince him to come along and help out. He's in his mid-twenties, I reckon. He's really big and muscly, with long lank hair pulled back in a ponytail. He looks like some band's roadie. Justine is only nineteen, but she's been a professional singer and songwriter since she was sixteen. She went to some posh drama and dance school in London but is now at the music college in Salford to train to become a voice coach.

She's stunning: black and tall, with the most amazing figure. She saw an ad asking for volunteers up in the common room at the college, so she decided to come along, and even brought her mate Dave with her. He's a keyboard player and programmer. He's got a shiny bald head and loads of piercings.

I'm the youngest and most inexperienced out of all of them, and I was convinced I was going to make a complete fool of myself. Suddenly the safe confines of my damp old garage seemed very appealing, and I wished I could just go back there and pretend that I'd never agreed to this whole thing.

Salford Music College was giving us a rehearsal studio for free and providing us with a load of equipment, so we all caught a bus over there. We were just a handful of devotees, because a lot of people had dropped out, preferring to do other stuff like sport instead. Ellie, of course, was up for it. She was raring to sing her lungs out. Emma and Shula, who had become inseparable, were in, and there was Rafi, who lives entirely in a world of hard-core American rap and is convinced he's P. Diddy's long-lost brother, and Benjamin and Dotun, whom I didn't know anything about but who said they were keen to muck around with some samplers and see what we were up to.

There was a buzz of excitement on the bus. Ellie was trying to coax Justine into giving us all a song. She eventually agreed to, but in true professional style explained that she would have to do some exercises first to warm up. She began some scales, demonstrating her amazing vocal range, but her voice cracked at one point and she spluttered to a halt. Coughing and clasping her throat, she reached for some water from her bag.

Everyone was silent as they looked on with concern, but out of the silence came Ellie, brandishing a packet of throat sweets that she'd magicked out of thin air and proclaiming: "The show must go on!" Ellie had been practicing harmonies with Emma all morning and was so excited about the opportunity of receiving training from people who knew what they were doing that she wasn't about to let anything spoil it. She practically forced a throat sweet down Justine's neck.

When we got to the music college, we decided that for the first session we should just concentrate on introducing the group to all of the instruments, getting them involved in a bit of drumming, singing, and so on and developing it from there. Everyone sat in a circle and the four of us went round and demonstrated what we could do. I didn't slip up once and managed to get through my turn without falling off my seat from nerves.

Afterward, everyone rotated round the room and did something different. The noise was incredible, but the atmosphere was good. We were all fired up. Rafi even plucked out a few chords on the guitar, which was a minor miracle seeing as only half an hour earlier he had declared guitar music "dead and buried and gone to rock heaven." Shula seemed most interested in the drums; she had the right rhythm for them. She watched my every move and got really frustrated when she'd get things wrong. Justine had the entire group in the palms of her hands with her cool moves and deep soul voice. Ellie just watched in awe. I tried to imagine her when she was little, growing up in the back rooms of clubs, listening to her mum belt out her set night after night, and I thought how silent her life must seem now. Perhaps the music group was helping to fill that void.

After a couple of hours I popped out of the music room to go to the toilet. I was feeling pretty pleased with myself and how the workshop was going, and there was a rush of adrenaline surging through me. I was practically skipping to the toilet and had just turned the corner from our studio when I banged straight into Darren. I couldn't believe my eyes.

"Leyla, what are you doing here?" He leant over and kissed me on the lips.

"What are *you* doing here more like?" I was in shock. I checked over my shoulder to see if anyone from our group had followed me out of the room to go to the toilet as well.

"I told you, I'm doing my guitar exams this month. My teacher is based at this college. I've been coming here every week for the past month in the lead-up to my exams."

"I didn't realize it was this college."

"Yeah, it is. What are you up to anyway, looking shifty, hovering around the corridors?"

"I don't look shifty, do I?" I leant against the wall and tried to look as relaxed as possible, even though my heart was going like the clappers. "I'm just here for that music workshop I told you about. I'm giving some drumming lessons and stuff like that, you know."

"Brilliant. I've got a break now—can I come and sit in on a session? I'd love to see you in action."

"No," I said, a little too quickly.

"What do you mean? People are always ducking in and out of music workshops in this place. Come on, don't be shy."

"No. I mean, it's our policy not to let anyone into the group. Everyone's a learner, and having an audience could be really off-putting and intimidating during the first few sessions. We want them to feel completely relaxed. You know how it is when you're starting out. It can be really embarrassing."

"Hmm, I suppose. I'd still love to see you play, though."

"You will one day, I promise. Just not today, okay?"

"There are loads of people around today. It was hard to find a studio. Mikey, my teacher, said that they were loaning one of the big rooms out to some hospital that was setting up some sort of music group for kids who are ill. I was in hospital for a week when I was eight with appendicitis and nearly died of boredom and malnutrition, so God knows how some of them who have been in there for months on end must feel."

"Ah, bless. I didn't realize you were such a kind and caring soul, Darren," I teased, giving his cheek a quick squeeze and ruffling his hair. "Listen, I've got to get back. I've been out here ages; they'll be wondering where I've got to."

"Okay. What are you doing later? We could go out somewhere, do something." He grabbed me by the hips and pulled me toward him. I could have stayed there forever, but suddenly panicked that Emma would come out looking for me and there'd be a lot of explaining to do.

"I'll call you when I get home. I've really got to go. I'll see you later, okay?" I ran off to the toilets and locked myself in a cubicle, slumping down on the toilet seat. I had to give Darren time to get back to his own room without seeing me go into the big studio where the kids from the "hospital" were playing. I knew that he'd ask too many questions and it would all get very complicated. I had to go back in the room and forget I'd even seen him. I could worry about the implications of him finding anything out another time.

After we'd wrapped things up at the music college, Emma

and I went home to her place. She said that her mum was out on a works do and she didn't fancy being in the flat all on her own. I thought about the vague plans I'd made to see Darren, but decided that I could give him a call and arrange to meet him the next day. I was feeling pretty tired anyway and wasn't really up to doing anything other than slobbing in front of the telly. I decided not to mention to Emma that I'd bumped into Darren because I knew that she'd worry too much. She had enough on her plate as it was, and it didn't seem worth it. He wouldn't be going to the college for much longer, because his exams were coming up really soon, and so he wouldn't necessarily find out anything anyway.

Emma looked a bit drawn later on in the evening. She'd been in top form all day—singing her heart out, bossing people around, and generally acting like she was behind the scenes of a West End musical—but when we got home she went straight to her room and flopped down on her bed. I fell asleep on the beanbag in her room, then woke up when her watch alarm went off. Emma dragged herself reluctantly off the bed, tutting. She came back a few minutes later carrying a plateful of sandwiches and a pot of yogurt under her arm.

"I'm still bloated after all the food we had at the center. Are you hungry already?" I asked, slapping my full belly.

"No, not really. It's just time for my tablets and I've got to take them with food or else I'm sick as a dog." Emma put the tray down and knelt on the floor to rummage around under her bed. She pulled a big plastic box out and opened it up. There must have been about twenty different packets and bottles of pills in there. I was shocked to see so many. It looked like a pharmacy.

"Does Mrs. Granger know you've nicked half her dispensary supplies from downstairs?"

Emma didn't look up and seemed quiet and withdrawn. She sat on the edge of the bed and placed four different tablets on the rim of the sandwich plate.

"Mmm, looks tasty, doesn't it? 'Would you like mayo with those pills, madam?'" she said, mock-waiter style, and stared blankly down at the tray of food. She nibbled on a tuna sandwich, tearing off the crusts, then slinging them onto the tray.

"Why do you keep them under the bed, Em?" I asked.

"Can you imagine Jo and Lucia looking in my drawers for makeup or whatever, like they do, and finding enough drugs to start up a branch of Boots? I'm not risking it. They're always snooping around. It's hard enough with them asking me where I get off to when I go for my checkups at the hospital."

"How often do you have to take them then?"

"It feels like every half an hour. I'm like a robot. My alarm goes off and no matter what I'm doing I've got to stop and take my tablets."

"How do you get away with it at college?" I was curious.

"Oh, I take them first thing in the morning, then when I get home at about fourish and then later in the night, about now."

"Do you have to eat every time?"

"No, only with certain kinds."

"So what do they do exactly?" I quizzed her.

"Oh God, I don't know. I'm a bit down about taking them at the moment. Apparently they reduce the level of virus in the blood, what they call the viral load, and slow down the destruction of the immune system so that my ability to fight infections will improve. That's the textbook answer, at least."

"They can only be doing you good then, Em. Is it some sort of combination treatment you're on? I saw something about it on the telly the other day. They reckon it's as near as you can get to a cure for HIV, don't they? It's worked miracles for some people. There was this one guy being interviewed who was saying that he was really, really ill, practically on the brink of death, and he went to America and was told about this combination therapy. Within a few months of being on the treatment he felt like a new man. He was going on about how the virus in his system was virtually undetectable and that the illness was under control. So you've got to keep taking them, Em, they're good for you."

"I bet the program didn't tell you about all the different side effects, though, and the fact that for some people the treatment doesn't work at all. People go through hell taking up to thirty tablets a day, have chronic diarrhea, nausea, headaches, pins and needles for weeks on end, and then there's no guarantee the pills are going to work. I bet they didn't tell you all that, did they?"

"But they reckon these drugs have improved the lives of thousands of people with HIV. Okay, I don't know all the facts, but I've heard that doctors are more optimistic that HIV-positive people can live normal lives for much longer because of this treatment."

"Do you call this normal? Setting my alarm to go off three times a day so I can guzzle down a fistful of drugs that make me shit myself like a baby? With every prescription dished out they should supply nappies."

Emma tore at the sandwiches on her plate, breaking each one into tiny little pieces.

"Ugh, that's gross. But, Em, come on, you've only just

started taking them. It must be a shock to the system at first. You're bound to get used to the routine."

"Will I? I don't know anymore. I didn't feel ill until I started taking these drugs. My doctor told me that if I started this combination therapy as soon as possible it would improve my life chances dramatically. He told me all this in front of my mum, and after that she was calling them 'miracle drugs,' falling over herself to get me my first prescription. It seemed to give her some hope, but it's not her who's got to take the bloody things."

She took the last pill with a swig of orange juice, scrunching up her face as she did so. "Yeuch," she said, wiping her mouth with the back of her hand. "Anyway, I don't always take them. I can't be arsed. Mum can't force me. How would *she* like it? I'm not even ill. Missing one or two pills isn't going to kill me."

I knew how much I hated taking any sort of medicine and that to have to take them three times a day to a strict timetable had to be awful. But the alternative was worse, in my eyes. To stop taking them and allow the illness to run its course seemed a horrific option, whereas if Emma took the drugs there was a chance that the virus could be kept under control for years. I could totally understand why her mum was putting so much pressure on her to continue the treatment; the alternative was too painful to even contemplate. "I don't want to see you get ill, Em," I said.

"I know, I know. It's just I've got to weigh up all the pros and cons. At the moment the side effects and having to take the pills wherever I am, no matter what I'm doing, are *big* cons, and there aren't many pros. And there's no guarantee that they're going to work anyway."

Emma sighed heavily before continuing. "Mum found a stash of the pills I hadn't taken the other day and she practically had a nervous breakdown. I'd hidden them, but she caught me out. She knows more about the treatments than I do and she reckons that they'll never work if I don't stick to them properly and take them every day. So I've promised her that I'll take them for a year and then see how I'm getting on. If I'm still struggling with the regime and suffering from awful side effects, then no matter what my viral load is I'm not going to stay on the treatment just for everyone else's sake. If it's making me miserable and depressed, it's just not worth it."

I could see how determined she was to keep control of her own life and her own body. Even though we all wanted the best for her, it was her life, and only she could decide what to do with it. It seemed so easy from our point of view just to take the drugs unquestioningly, but to be as brave as Emma and look at it from the perspective that it might not actually make her happy in the long run was an attitude that I had to admire. "So, Em, if you hadn't started taking any drugs at all, would you be really ill by now or what?" I asked.

"No, not necessarily. It affects people differently. Some people don't notice any change to their health for years and years. I could be totally fit and healthy for ages. Others might have weaker immune systems or something and they can become ill early on and might suffer some sort of serious infection. You can still get treated for it—take antibiotics and stuff; you won't die or anything. I read somewhere the other day that on average it takes about ten years for HIV to progress to full-blown AIDS if you're not on any sort of treatment."

"And what if you are on treatment?"

"They don't know yet. Not enough people have been on medication long enough for anyone to know how long HIV-positive people can live."

"Please stay well, Em. I couldn't bear it if anything happened to you."

ELEVEN

IT WAS FRIDAY NIGHT AND DARREN HAD INVITED ME and Sarah to a house party that one of his friends was having not far from where Darren lived. This guy's parents had gone away for a long weekend, taking his younger sister with them and leaving him in charge of the house. Big mistake!

Every parent in the world should know that if they go away on holiday and leave their seventeen-year-old son on his own in the house then he's going to have a party. I'm sorry, but it's practically a child's right to trash their parents' house at least once in their lifetime. But the parents always come home, find their drinks cabinet empty and half their kitchen demolished, and then act shocked. I mean, "Urrmm, hel-looo." I remember being forced to go away with my parents to Derbyshire for a week when I was thirteen while Sadie stayed at home. I asked her if she was going to have a party while we were away and she went and told Mum what I'd said. I got into trouble for entertaining the idea on her behalf and Sadie got a gold star and walked away polishing her halo. They've never left me alone in the house since that one time I even dared to *think* of having a party in their absence.

I was looking forward to the night's shenanigans. House parties were always the best and I was excited about spending some time with Darren. We only ever saw each other briefly at school, down at Georgio's, or at the occasional party like this one.

I walked over to Sarah's at about seven thirty to pick her up. As per usual she wasn't ready, so her mum waved me inside. I bounded up the stairs, past the Virgin Marys and pictures of Jesus, straight into Sarah's room and found her on all fours on the floor with her bum in the air. She was wearing a pair of black trousers but only a bra on top.

"What you looking for?" I said loudly, knowing that she hadn't heard me come in.

She jumped up, looking shocked and covering her chest with her arms. "I wish you'd bloody knock. You frighten the life out of me every time you barge in here."

"What are you doing scrabbling around on the floor with just your bra on?"

"I've lost it. I had it a minute ago. I was just putting it in and it bounced out of my hand. It's got to be here somewhere." Her eyes scanned the room in desperation.

"What? What have you lost?" I demanded.

"Ahem, isn't it obvious?" she said, thrusting out her chest and looking down at her boobs.

I studied her chest and noticed that one boob was in fact bigger than the other and that she looked slightly off balance.

"Are you saying that you've lost a breast or what?"

"Well, in a manner of speaking, yes."

"Listen, Sarah, what's going on? You had two tits the last time I saw you, and that was only yesterday. It can't have disappeared overnight."

"No, stupid, my fake breast." She reached down inside her bra and pulled out a soft, wobbly, flesh-colored sac that looked like a piece of uncooked chicken. "I've lost the other one of these."

"Oh my God, I didn't know you had false tits." I fell back onto her bed in shock. "How long have you had them?"

"Only a week, for God's sake. I got them last weekend while you were at your workshop. They're fantastic. Cheaper than a boob job and a lot less hassle. If you don't lose them, that is." She gestured for me to have a feel of the chicken thing in her hand. I gave it a prod with my finger, but that's as far as I went.

"I'm never sure what I'm going to find when I walk in this room. One week you're wrapped in cling film, the next you're shoving freaky pieces of poultry down your bra. Are you really that worried about your body? You're absolutely gorgeous as you are."

"They are a bit weird, aren't they?" We both started giggling at the sight of the thing wobbling in Sarah's hands. "Maybe I could serve it up on a doily as a delicacy for the party."

"It's such a waste of time trying to look like all those models in the magazines," I told her. "If you gave me five thousand pounds a week I could look that amazing all the time as well, but even then I'm not sure I'd want to be that skinny. I couldn't handle smoking a fag instead of having lunch, or eating a carrot for my tea. I'm happy the way I am, and so should you be."

"I saw Emma in town the other day. She's looking dead skinny. It's her you should be lecturing, not me. She's going for the waif image, big style." Sarah sucked in her cheeks to mimic how gaunt Emma's face looked.

Sarah's words stung, but she had no idea that she could possibly be hurting me. She was right—Emma had lost a lot of weight—but I couldn't tell her the reasons why, even though I wanted to so badly. I wanted to spill it all out there and then and tell Sarah how worried and how frightened I was that Em was going to get really ill and I wouldn't be able to cope. Tears sprang to my eyes, and I had to fight with myself to stop them from pouring down my cheeks; I thought that if I started crying I'd never stop. I pretended I had something in my eye and ran to the bathroom, telling Sarah to hurry up and find her missing mammary gland while I was in the toilet.

I emerged a few minutes later, composed and ready to get on with the evening. Sarah was faffing around putting glitter on her chest after having found her lost property.

"I suppose I can only be grateful you haven't gone under the knife yet," I tutted. "Get a move on. We're missing valuable party time."

The party was in full swing by the time we got there. As we walked up the road toward the noise, a police car drove slowly past, full of coppers ready to pounce at the slightest hint of a disturbance. We didn't need to ask which house it was. A strobe light flashed to the beat of a booming bass, and as we got nearer we could feel the vibrations of the blaring music under our feet. The house, ablaze with light and pulsating like it was alive, was stuck in the middle of a subdued suburban street. Sarah and I giggled at the thought of all the neighbors cowering on their sofas, trying to block out the noise as they attempted to watch their Friday night favorites on the telly.

There was a gang of lads hovering around the front door, smoking and laughing at one lad who was skidding down the slightly raised driveway in a supermarket trolley, crashing into the gate, wetting himself laughing, and then going back for more.

Inside, there were people everywhere: slouched over sofas, sat on top of the enormous amps, crowded round two guys who were DJing in one corner. A thick cloud of smoke shrouded the entire living room, which was full of people dancing and spilling drinks as they jumped to the music. It was absolutely packed, mostly with sixth-formers but with a couple of people from our year as well. The big French doors leading out to the back garden had steamed up, and people had written messages on the glass. When we walked in, one guy was busy writing "My mother made me a homosexual" in the steam, and Sarah rushed over and wrote underneath, "Can she make me a woolly jumper?" I dragged her off to the kitchen before she got up to any more mischief, and we searched for something to drink. I recognized Jimmy, whose party it was, crouched down on the floor. Darren had introduced me to him in school so that I wouldn't feel so awkward about just turning up at his party. He was brushing up a smashed glass, so I knelt down and said hi.

"Oh, hi. God, this is a nightmare," he said, his voice tight with worry. "The party only started about an hour ago and I've already lost count of all the glasses that have been smashed. More people than I thought have come. My mum is going to kill me."

"They say you never enjoy your own party—it's too stressful."

"I wish somebody had told me that before half of Bury descended on the place."

A lad with shaggy Oasis-type hair, a Ben Sherman shirt, and baggy jeans came up to Jimmy and put his arm around him. "Chill, man. It's a cool party. You need a toke on this." He passed Jimmy a spliff. Jimmy smiled and leant back against the cooker to enjoy his smoke.

He passed it to me, but I decided not to. Grass made me paranoid, and I wanted to be in top form for when I saw Darren. I was just about to go and have a look for him when a girl came flying into the kitchen clutching a pint glass full of a mysterious dark-brown concoction.

"They've dared me to down this pint of shorts. I thought I'd better be near a sink. It's got everything in it: Malibu, tequila, sherry. Here goes." She raised her glass, tipped back her head, and swilled the weird-looking mixture down her throat. She'd drunk half a pint when she spluttered to a halt and ran out the back door with her hand to her mouth, muttering that she was going to be sick.

"Where did you get all the shorts from?" Jimmy yelled.

"The drinks cabinet in there." She pointed toward the dining room.

Jimmy sat down on the breakfast bar stool and put his head in his hands. "My parents are going to murder me."

I patted him on the back, comforting him halfheartedly, but I'd decided that I'd had enough of regretful hosts and needed to find someone who was in the party mood. Sarah was nowhere to be seen, so I decided to have a wander around to see if I could spot Darren. I recognized a couple of Darren's friends, who were chatting on the stairs. They said that they'd last seen him upstairs in the bathroom announcing into a bog brush that all the action at a house party always took place in the toilet, so he was staying where the action was and no one was to attempt to remove him.

I wandered on up and opened the bathroom door.

Darren was lying fully clothed in the bath, clutching a can of beer, and singing into a hairbrush; I was relieved that he'd ditched the bog brush for a slightly classier model of mike. The bathroom was completely empty and totally devoid of all action. Darren raised his can of beer when he saw me, and a huge grin broke out across his face.

"I've come looking for the action," I said with a cheeky smile.

"Then you've come to the right place, baby." Darren pushed himself up with his elbows and lunged forward, grabbing me by the arm and pulling me on top of him. He always made me feel excited. I was tingling all over. "You're looking as gorgeous as ever," he said, and pulled me closer so that he could kiss me.

We'd been kissing for a while when I felt Darren's hand move down to my breasts. It felt nice and I felt comfortable and happy to be with him, so I didn't protest. He was struggling to open my bra, so I helped him out, and felt the goose bumps rise all over me as he placed his hands on my bare breasts. I felt the bulge between his legs as he pressed his groin against my thigh, and I kissed him harder. I knew that I wanted this. I felt so close to him, so right with him. No bloke had ever made me feel so good before.

Darren whispered in my ear, telling me to leave the bath. We heaved ourselves out and stood facing each other. Darren began to undress me. I felt shy but exhilarated, ready for him but scared. Conflicting emotions crowded my head so that I couldn't think straight, but I just knew in my gut and in my heart that I wanted to be with him. As we undressed each other, Darren kissed me from my neck to my toes, stopping to play with my belly-button ring with his tongue. We sank down onto the bathroom floor together in a firm embrace. He put his face close to mine, then asked me gently if I wanted to have sex.

I couldn't speak. I'd come close to having sex before, but it hadn't felt like this. This was different—it felt so special. I'd never been so full of emotion. Darren was making me feel more alive than I'd ever been in my life. I nodded and had just reached out to put his beautiful face in my hands when suddenly the bathroom door, which we were lying up against, jerked open an inch as someone attempted to come in. I scrambled for a towel with which to cover myself as Darren leapt to his feet, lurching for the lock.

"I thought you'd locked it."

"When did I get the chance? You pulled me on top of you the second I walked in here." I was trembling a little as I stood there in the towel.

"Well, it's locked now. No one can get in. Come here," he said, reaching for my arm to bring me close to him again. "Don't let that spoil the moment. Let's pretend we were never interrupted."

But the moment *had* been broken, and suddenly I wasn't so wrapped up in such intense emotion anymore and was able to think straight. "What about a condom? Have you got any?"

"Uh, no, but we can be careful. I'll, you know, pull out before I go too far. It'll be fine. Don't you want to do it anymore?"

"No, it's not that, it's just we *have* to use a condom."

Darren looked in the cabinet above the sink and in the small chest of drawers next to the bath, but couldn't find any condoms. "I don't reckon Jimmy's parents see much action between the sheets these days." He sighed and slid down onto the floor where his clothes were.

I went over to him and stroked his back cautiously. I stuttered and opened my mouth to say something, but couldn't get the words out. After we'd been so intimate only a few minutes before, suddenly Darren felt like a stranger. What had been a perfectly relaxed atmosphere was now tense and awkward. I wanted our stolen moment back. I had to say something to save the situation, but I was completely unsure of how he was going to react—I couldn't read his face.

"Look, Darren, it's not that I don't want to be with you, because I do. I really like you. You make me feel fantastic. I've just promised myself never to have sex without a condom. I'd hate myself if I was stupid enough to get carried away and not be careful." I held my breath, waiting for him to respond. I was so scared that I'd ruined everything between us, but at the same time I knew I was right. God knows, I understood what the consequences of unsafe sex could be.

He pulled his T-shirt back on and looked hurt and disappointed. I felt totally deflated and just as cheated as he did, but I needed him to say something to reassure me that everything was okay, that he understood.

He spent ages looking at me, really looking at me, then eventually spoke. "You're so different from all the other girls

I know. You make me feel really intense. I really feel and think deeply about things when I'm with you." He put his arm around my shoulder. "I want to roll about this bathroom floor with you all night, but I respect what you're saying. I know it's stupid not to use a condom—it's just easier not to, isn't it? But you don't want to get pregnant and ruin your great drumming career, now do you?" He stood up and jumped into his trousers.

"We don't have to go, though. We can stay in here longer if you want." I was still unsure as to how exactly he was feeling, and I just wanted him to hold me and make me feel secure.

"No. Come on, let's go and find out what's going on downstairs. Are you going down in that towel or were you planning on putting your clothes back on?"

As I got back into my clothes, I thought about how relieved I was that at least Darren hadn't turned into a slithering cold fish as soon as he realized that he wasn't going to be getting his leg over that night. There weren't many boys his age who would be quite so understanding, I knew. Most lads were just after a shag, and if they didn't get it then a girl was history.

But I was also relieved that we'd been interrupted when we were. If we hadn't suddenly been jolted out of that intense situation, I wasn't sure whether I would have had the guts to stop what Darren and I were doing to ask if he had a condom. And that was worrisome. Before tonight I was sure that I was responsible and sensible enough to stay aware and in control at all times, but I now saw that the reality was very different. I thought about Emma and realized how easy it was to get swept along and to lose your head. It could happen to anyone;

it was as simple as that. How anyone could judge Emma for what had happened to her, I didn't know. There were hundreds of girls in my school alone who had done exactly the same thing as Emma; they had just been lucky enough not to get caught out.

Darren was sat quietly on the toilet, and when I told him I was ready he stood up and told me I looked stunning. I wasn't really in the party mood anymore, but I wasn't ready to leave Darren either. I followed him down the stairs, where a gang of his mates were still sat drinking. They'd obviously figured out that we'd been in the bathroom together and had heard all the fuss when someone had tried to get in there. We were treated to a barrage of jeers and taunts as we weaved our way between them: "Weyhey, on ya, Dazza" and "Get in there, my son" and "Give her one from me next time." They made me feel cheap and dirty, as though our intimacy was suddenly public property that they could laugh and leer at. The warm, special feeling that I held inside me was slowly fading in the cold light of their gross remarks.

I wanted Darren to say something to them, to tell them that I was more than just a quick shag on the bathroom floor, but he just kept on walking as if he hadn't heard them. I couldn't let them get away with it. I knew they'd laugh and get defensive at any retaliation, but I couldn't just walk on by. I stopped before I reached the bottom of the stairs and, turning to face them with a cool and calm glare, said, "Your brains aren't big enough to even begin to comprehend what went on in that bathroom, and your balls certainly aren't big enough to do what Darren did for me tonight." And with that, I turned on my heel and headed for the living room. None of them said anything until I was just through the door, and then I heard one of them murmur "Stupid bitch" before asking his mate to pass him another can of beer.

A few days later I was stood shivering in my shorts and T-shirt on the school netball court again. I was so cold I decided to actually put some effort into the game for once, just to keep myself warm. Claire Higgins and her cronies were lurking about the corners of the court, whispering and laughing and casting filthy looks at anyone who wasn't in their gang. They were so pathetic they made me laugh; they probably couldn't even go to the toilet without one another.

I was glad I was concentrating on the netball rather than getting angry about them. But because I was focusing so intently on the game, I didn't notice Claire Higgins sneak up beside me and stick her foot out to trip me up just as I was running to catch a particularly high ball. I landed on the tarmac court with a thud and felt my right knee take the full blow of my fall. Blood gushed everywhere, and I felt faint at the sight of it. Mrs. Rose, our PE teacher, rushed over and crouched down at my side to get a good look at my knee, but just as she moved to pull my leg straight Claire Higgins shouted out, "Don't touch her, miss, you'll catch AIDS."

Without thinking about my next move for even one second, I was up on my feet, with blood dripping down my shin, racing after Claire across the courts. I'd caught her off guard, as she hadn't expected me to leap off the ground, so she didn't have much of a head start and I managed to grab her by her jumper and push her against the fence. I swung her round and slapped her hard across the face and, in shock, she fell to the ground in a crumpled heap.

I was in shock too over my own actions. I'd never hit

anyone before in my whole life—well, except for my sister—but now I'd actually managed to floor the hardest girl in our year. All of Claire's hangers-on gathered round her, cooing and comforting her, asking if there was anything they could do. Pathetic. A red-faced Mrs. Rose brought up the rear, demanding an explanation. The pain in my knee was excruciating after the extra exertion I'd put on it. When neither of us answered because we were too wrapped up in our pain and injuries, Mrs. Rose grabbed us both by the wrists and marched us to the headmaster.

Sat outside Mr. Strong's office, I had time to calm down and think clearly about what had just happened. Either Claire knew that HIV and AIDS was an issue in my life and had found something out about Em, or it was just her latest way of grinding her victims down—by telling people that so-and-so had AIDS, the same way she went around telling people that so-and-so was a lesbian or so-and-so's mum was an alcoholic. I decided to wait to hear her explanation before trying to justify my reaction—I didn't want to let something slip about why Claire had hit a very raw nerve. Either way, I didn't regret laying into her. Claire Higgins had it coming to her. Even if the AIDS thing was just her latest taunt, it proved how low she was capable of going in her mission to instill fear and misery in anyone who wasn't a member of her nasty little entourage. She deserved all she got.

Mr. Strong called us into his office and asked us to sit down. He was sat in a big leather swivel chair with his back to us. All we could see was his bald head poking over the top. He left us to stew in silence for a while before swinging round to face us. It was no surprise to find him wearing the same navy blue suit he'd worn every day since I'd been at Bishops High. It was shiny from so much wear, and dandruff speckled his shoulders.

Mrs. Rose explained what had happened while Mr. Strong listened, pulling on the whiskers of a stuffed fox on the windowsill the whole time she spoke. When she had finished Mr. Strong demanded an explanation from us both. Neither of us spoke, until he said that if either of us had any plans to go on the school trip to Venice the following term we could think again, because he was withdrawing all privileges immediately. It was at that point that Claire Higgins started talking. She'd been talking about going to Venice for months and had been boasting about all the new clothes her parents had bought her for the trip. She had too much to lose, and so she started spilling the beans.

"I was only trying to protect Mrs. Rose, sir. My brother is in Leyla's boyfriend's class and he told me that Leyla's been hanging around with people who have AIDS, and when I saw that Leyla was bleeding I didn't want Mrs. Rose to touch her blood, just in case she caught something. I was only thinking of Mrs. Rose, sir. Leyla went for me like a madwoman."

"But it was you who tripped me up in the first place," I snarled at her.

"I was trying to get the ball. It was a game of netball, remember. People get tangled up all the time."

"Whatever the case, Claire, do you really think that such an over-the-top reaction was appropriate when you saw that Leyla was bleeding?" Mr. Strong said, straightening out his brown nylon tie. "You know that we do not stand for bullying in this school."

"Oh, so you want Mrs. Rose to catch AIDS then, do you? Well, excuse me for trying to help."

"Look, Claire, you can leave your soap-opera melodrama

at home. I don't know what information you've heard about Leyla, but I will not tolerate idle gossip in my school. I suggest—no, I demand—that you apologize to Leyla immediately."

"But, sir, it was her who belted me. She's the one who should be apologizing to me. It's not fair," she said petulantly.

"I do not condone Leyla's actions in any way and would like her to apologize to you in due course, but I do feel that this whole situation has arisen as a result of the taunts and gibes that you are continually hurling at your fellow classmates. Your behavior does not go unnoticed, and from now on I shall be taking harsh measures to ensure that no pupil of mine suffers under you. I will be informing your parents that you will be unable to go on the school trip and that all privileges have been suspended until further notice."

"But sir. Oh my God, you can't. I *have* to go on that trip. You can't stop me. This isn't fair. She beats me up and I'm the one getting punished. My parents won't stand for this, you know."

Claire Higgins was on her feet. Her face was purple and she looked as though she was going to blow a gasket any second. Mrs. Rose was asked to remove her from the head's office. I couldn't help but smile, witnessing Claire Higgins get her comeuppance once and for all, but the smile was wiped from my face when Mr. Strong asked me to apologize to her before she left the room. The words stuck in my throat. I couldn't quite bring myself to say "Sorry" to her. But the longer the silence in the room drew out the more painful I knew it would be to say the words, so I sat up straight in my chair, looked her in the eye, and said that I was sorry for hitting her.

"Yeah, and I'll be sending you the medical bills. This isn't the end of this, you know," she threatened, with a look of true hatred in her eye that made me shudder all over. I got up to leave, but Mr. Strong asked me to stay to answer a few more questions. "You were wrong to hit Claire, and I hope that I don't see a repeat performance of your appalling behavior ever again. But I am also concerned about the root of Claire's taunts today. She was dealing with a very serious issue, one that I feel needs to be addressed. Do you want to tell me why she chose to taunt you with as grave a subject as AIDS in the first place?"

"No, not really." I didn't want to have to tell him anything. I was so worried about protecting Emma that I thought the less I said the better.

"Leyla, you do understand how serious an issue this is. If there is anything you can do to help me understand the situation a little better, so as to ensure that such malicious gossip is brought to an abrupt halt, it would be greatly appreciated."

He seemed to be quite sympathetic, and he *had* stuck up for me in front of Claire Higgins. Maybe I could open up to him a little bit, to see if we could somehow make a difference to how people in the school felt about HIV and AIDS. I mulled it over in my head and decided to tell him something about the Saturday workshops. I wouldn't have to mention Emma at all.

"It's just that . . . you know I play the drums," I started off hesitantly. "Well, I've started giving some other kids drumming lessons on Saturdays and they're all from this support center for people living with or affected by HIV and AIDS. It's like a charity, and I'm helping out a bit. Somebody must have found out about what I'm doing, and Claire is always the first to hear, so she goes to the extreme of thinking I've now got HIV and am therefore going to be infecting the entire school."

"I see, I see." Mr. Strong swiveled on his chair, nodding his head.

"So that's all there is to it, sir. Do you think we could do a special assembly on HIV or something like that? We could get someone in to give a talk so that some of the myths about HIV are dispelled—then more people would be able to put the Claire Higginses of this world in their place. Do you think that would be possible, sir?" I was quite fired up by the idea and excited to have someone in authority, someone who might be able to help, on my side.

Mr. Strong was rubbing his chin, a concerned look on his face. "Mmm, we'll have to see about that. It's a very sensitive subject. I'd have to think about it carefully." Then he slapped his legs and jumped to his feet. "Thank you, Leyla. You may go now."

When I got home from school that evening Mum and Dad were sat at the kitchen table, not talking, just sat there with serious expressions on their faces. At first I thought something bad had happened, like someone had died or something, but it didn't take me long to figure out that they'd heard about what had happened at school and I was in for a lecture. It was the last thing I needed, so I tried to get past them without seeming too concerned about the fact that they were obviously waiting for me.

Dad stopped me before I could leave the room. "Just a minute, Leyla, your mum and I want to have a word with you. Come and sit down."

"Oh, Dad, I've got loads of homework to do. Is this going

to take long?" I whined as I dragged myself to the table.

"I don't know, Leyla. We just want to ask you a few questions, that's all."

Then it was Mum's turn. "We've had a call from Mr. Strong, your headmaster, who sounded very concerned about you. Something about a bullying incident on the netball court today. He attempted to explain why it all came about in the first place, but that's the bit we don't really understand. We thought you might be able to shed some light on it for us."

Mum was trying to remain calm, but there was a suppressed, threatening tone in her voice as well. Reading between the lines, I knew that what she really wanted to say was: "What the hell does your headmaster mean when he says that you've been working for some bloody AIDS charity that we know absolutely nothing about? You'd better have a bloody good explanation or you're in for a battering, young lady." But her and Dad had obviously had a chat before I'd arrived home, to discuss how they were going to try to handle the situation with a calm approach.

"Shed light on what, Mum? Some stupid bully at school trips me up, rambles on about a load of offensive crap, I lose it and go for her jugular. There's nothing more to tell. She had it coming to her. She's always picking on someone or other. I just lost my temper today and gave her a taste of her own medicine."

"Leyla, she's been in your class for five years, and you've never let her bother you before. There must be more to it than that. What's going on, Leyla? What's all this stuff about AIDS and some place you've been going to on Saturdays? I sounded like a right fool on the phone to Mr. Strong. I was adamant that you were going to some music workshop that had been organized by your music teacher. Mr. Strong hadn't heard anything about it and said that you'd told him yourself that you were giving lessons to some kids with AIDS or something." Mum gave a long, weary sigh and looked at me sternly. "Leyla, you've been lying to us, and we want to know what's going on."

"Why does Mr. Strong have to go sticking his nose in? It's none of his business."

"He's just trying to clamp down on bullying in the school. He's also concerned about this AIDS business. He's wondering, just as we are, if you know what you're doing, getting involved with those . . . sort of people." The way she said "those sort of people" made me want to scream, but at this point I realized I would have to tell them some of the truth before things got blown out of all proportion and got really messy. Nobody knew anything about Emma, and that's the way I wanted it to stay. If I told them the truth about the group it would explain a few things and I wouldn't have to tell them any more than that.

"Okay, okay. I'm sorry I lied to you, but I knew you wouldn't approve or would try to stop me, so I thought it would be easier just to get on with it and not get you involved. And anyway, I wasn't telling you complete lies—it *is* a music workshop that I've been going to. It's just that it's with a group who give support to children and families affected by HIV one way or another. They do different activities with the kids, and one of them is a music workshop that I'm helping out with because I can play the drums."

"So it's like a charity then, is it, and you're a volunteer?" Dad had been silent for a while, but his ears had suddenly pricked up. I misinterpreted his question as a sign of interest;

when I told him that yes, I was a volunteer, and enthusiastically talked a bit about what I did, he tutted and shook his head. "Well, charity begins at home, and we're not made of money, you know. You could be out earning your own pocket money every Saturday instead of coming to us the whole time asking for handouts left, right, and center. You can't afford to go volunteering your services."

They'd managed to keep up the cool, calm, rational approach for all of thirty seconds. I knew it was time for them to take the gloves off.

"Oh, Jeremy, all you think about is money. What about the fact that our daughter has been spending her Saturdays dealing with people who have got AIDS?" Mum practically spat out the word, like she was going to get infected just by mentioning it.

"Mum, there are children there younger than me who are HIV positive. How can you possibly talk about AIDS with such a look of disgust on your face? They're just ill, like any other kids with cancer or whatever."

"But, Leyla, do you . . . you know . . . come into *physical contact* with these children?"

"No, I'm placed with my drums in an airtight Perspex box in one corner of the room and they stand around outside and learn from there. That way I don't have to breathe the same air as them."

Mum hesitated for a moment, thinking about what I'd just said. "Okay, no need to be sarcastic. I'm just worried for you. It's a highly infectious disease, Leyla; I don't want you to be at risk. Nobody knows enough about the disease. You don't know what you're getting yourself into." She looked down at her hands for a while and then sat back in her seat, folding her arms defiantly in front of her. "Anyway, you're not going there again. We trusted you, Leyla. You lied to us and now you'll just have to accept the consequences."

I scraped back my chair from the table and stood up. I wasn't going to sit around in their company any longer. "This has got nothing to do with me lying to you, has it? I wasn't even lying really; I just left out a few details. This has got everything to do with your fear and ignorance. You're scared. It doesn't fit into the routine of things, does it? It's not quite normal, is it? I can't believe you're going to sit there and punish me for trying to do my bit to help. Why don't you practice what some of your stupid little messages scattered around the place tell you for once instead of just having them around the house for decoration." I pointed at a fridge magnet and read out the message: "'There have been times when you have had enough cares of your own and yet you cared.' You make me laugh. It's all just a show, isn't it? You're worse than I thought."

Dad moved to try and prevent me from leaving the room, but I dodged his grip and ran up the stairs three at a time, slamming my bedroom door behind me.

I'd been lying on my bed for half an hour, fuming, wondering how on earth I'd been spawned from such stupid parents, when the doorbell rang. I sat up and listened, praying that it was Sarah come to rescue me. I heard a male voice that I couldn't quite recognize, and could just make out Mum explaining that I'd been in a spot of bother at school and that she thought it was best I was left alone to calm down. I was too curious to find out who it was to stay in my room, so I sneaked to the top of the stairs to see who my mystery visitor was. Stood at the door, still in his school uniform, was Darren. I ran down to save him from Mum.

"I don't think it's a good idea that you have visitors tonight, dear," Mum said firmly.

"Mrs. Burgess, it's my fault Leyla got into trouble in the first place—me and my big mouth blabbing away to people about all sorts of things. I just want to apologize and get a few things straight. Just five minutes, please?"

Darren could charm the socks off anyone, and much to my surprise Mum agreed that he could stay for "half an hour and no longer." I showed him up to my room.

"I heard about what went off. I could kill that Claire Higgins. Are you hurt?" he asked.

"No, just fuming."

"Oh God, this is all my fault. I had history with Gareth Higgins, Claire Higgins's brother, first thing this morning, and we got chatting before break. Gareth works at the music college in Salford. He's just like a caretaker there on weekends, earning a bit of extra money. He said that he thought he'd seen you there last Saturday leaving with a group of people who were booked in as being from the hospital in town. Somebody at the college had mentioned to him that they were AIDS patients. So when he asked me if I knew that you went to the college, of course I said yes. Then this whole rumor, which Claire decided to spread, started that you had AIDS. I heard about it in the dinner hall at break. A gang of them were talking about how we'd been caught 'at it' in Jimmy's bathroom last Friday and that I should be careful if I didn't want to catch something. And then Claire goes and does that on the netball court."

"Who the hell do they think they are? I could kill them." I was angrier than ever. "Why would anyone with half a brain think that I'd have HIV or AIDS just because I'm in contact with people who are HIV positive? Not that that's even the point. How can anyone use something like AIDS to bully someone? Claire Higgins is the scum of the earth."

"So the group that you're doing music with *have* got AIDS then?"

"You've got nothing to worry about, you know. *I* haven't got it," I said defensively, not quite sure what Darren was thinking.

"I'm not bothered about that," Darren said softly.

He seemed genuinely shaken by the day's events. It was obvious he just wanted some answers to make sense of it all. I had to calm down and be straight with him. "Yeah, well, some of them are HIV positive, or someone in their family is, and they just go to this support group once a week. They've started up a music workshop and I go with them to the college to play the drums, and Claire Higgins thinks that's reason enough to go spouting off at school, thinking she can intimidate me. I only got so angry because I can see her ignorance infecting the entire school. Kids listen to people like Claire Higgins, you know. It's dangerous. She needs to be put in her place before she causes any more damage to people's lives."

We were both quiet then, Darren lost in thought and me still lost in my fury.

"You just keep on surprising me, Leyla. There's so much going on in there," he said, tapping me on the head. "I don't know where to start unraveling it all. There are not many girls your age who would give up their Saturdays to do something like that, you know."

I couldn't help thinking that if he knew about Emma it wouldn't seem quite so extraordinary to him, or to anyone else, for that matter. But of course I couldn't tell him that, and the undeserved respect he was suddenly paying me made me feel uncomfortable. "I'm not just being a Good Samaritan, you know. I get to play the drums in front of a live audience every week and fulfill my rock-legend fantasies." I laughed, desperate to lighten things up and move away from the issue. I was relieved that Darren had come round and helped fit the pieces of the jigsaw together—at least I knew that nothing had been linked back to Em. But I also felt a sense of doom, as though there could only be more trouble ahead. I sensed that this was just the beginning of a long and painful journey for the whole family.

"Leyla," Mum shouted from the bottom of the stairs. "Leyla, it's getting late. You can see your friend at school tomorrow."

Darren stood up to leave. "I'd better go. I just wanted to check that you were okay. I felt like shit when I heard what had happened. Just ignore all those idiots at school and let me know if there's any more trouble."

"My hero," I said mockingly, putting a limp wrist to my brow and swooning like a damsel in distress.

Darren laughed and shook his head. "You're unbelievable." I walked him to the front door and sneaked a quick kiss when I was sure Mum and Dad were safely in front of the box. Just before he left, he turned to me and said, "I know why you were so insistent about the condoms now."

"Sshh." I put my hand over his mouth and pushed him farther away from the house. "My mum doesn't miss a trick. She's had enough shocks for one night without hearing about her daughter's sex life, too."

"I just wanted to say sorry for being such a bonehead, thinking that we could just have sex like that. You can't be too careful, can you?"

"No, you can't." I smiled. "Listen, thanks for coming round. I'll see you in school tomorrow."

That night in bed I couldn't stop thinking about Emma and the gut feeling I had that I couldn't just sweep the day's events under the carpet and carry on as though nothing had happened. I decided that I'd have to tell her. I was worried sick about my mum and dad or anyone else finding out about her. She had a right to know, so that we could decide together what we were going to do.

At school the next day Mr. Strong asked our year to stay behind after assembly. Everyone shifted around in their seats, whispering to one another and wondering what it was all about. But I knew from the way Mr. Strong searched the room for my face in the crowd, then nodded to Mrs. Rose when he saw me, that it had something to do with yesterday's incident on the netball court.

Mr. Strong announced that Mrs. Rose was going to talk to us about some intimate issues to do with our lives as teenagers and then sat himself down behind the lectern and folded his arms. The room was deadly silent waiting for Mrs. Rose to begin. She was obviously nervous and embarrassed as she paced up and down in front of us.

"Now, I know a lot of you have had some sex education in biology classes, so I won't go into all the nitty-gritty about the birds and the bees." She smiled nervously and coughed into her hand. "What I *am* here to talk to you about are several issues to do with sex. As you all probably know, there are a number of infections and diseases you can catch from having unprotected sex, ranging from the more common and treatable infections to the terrible, incurable diseases that you really wouldn't want to live with. I'm sure most of you will have heard of thrush, herpes, chlamydia." A boy at the back of the hall shouted out "Genital warts" and everyone fell about laughing and whispering to one another until Mr. Strong stood up and demanded silence.

Mrs. Rose was now visibly flustered. "Umm, where was I? Ah yes, sexually transmitted diseases, or STDs for short. Along with the more common infections such as thrush, there is also the matter of contracting HIV if you are foolish enough to have unprotected sex. HIV is a very, very dangerous disease. It can be passed on to others through bodily fluids and will eventually develop into full-blown AIDS."

Mrs. Rose's voice was becoming deeper and more solemn, and she was drawing out every word. I could feel the whole room's eyes on me. Everyone had heard about what had happened the day before. I stared ahead, not moving a muscle.

"AIDS will kill you. It eats away at you until you eventually die a very sad and awful death." She paused dramatically, then straightened herself up and continued in a lighter tone. "Of course, it's a disease that mostly affects homosexuals or drug users—those people who share dirty needles—and the risk of a normal person getting it is still extremely low. But it is a danger nonetheless, and something for you to think about." She brushed herself down and smiled, becoming more and more relieved that the lecture was almost over. "I think what Mr. Strong and I want to say to you is *be safe*. Always wear a condom, or better still, don't have sex until you are in a steady relationship with a long-term partner, or wait until you are married. Thank you."

Mr. Strong dismissed us, and we all trooped out of the hall to our lessons. I was ready to blow, I was so angry. I thought Mr. Strong was going to consult me on doing a proper assembly about HIV and AIDS. I thought we were going to get some experts on HIV into the school to talk about it realistically, in a way that kids my age would listen to and understand. Instead they'd just rushed on in there without discussing it with anyone else, and they'd got it all wrong. They were so wrong. They couldn't possibly have been more wrong. Everyone in that hall, if they didn't know any better, would have left it thinking that they weren't at risk of contracting HIV, and would also have been wetting themselves laughing about what Mrs. Rose had said about not having sex before marriage. It was a joke.

I spent the rest of the day in a rage, and when the final bell rang I ran straight down to Emma's to tell her everything. I felt sick to my stomach just thinking about having to tell her. As I ran down the hill toward the flat, I thought how nice it would be to keep on running. I'd run straight out of Bury and keep on going until I found a place where no one knew me, where I would be left in peace to stare out at a vast horizon and slowly empty my mind.

That was it: I needed to slow down. My mind was racing at 100 miles an hour. I was functioning on nervous exhaustion. Slow down, slow down, I repeated to myself.

As I slowed to a walking pace, I got to Georgio's caff and looked in as I always did to check out who was in there from school. The usual mass of uniforms was there, like a swarm of buzzing bluebottles, but out of the corner of my eye I spotted someone who looked just like Emma from behind. I popped my head in the door to get a closer look. Emma was sat there with a coffee in front of her, happily chatting away to Gary, the friend of Darren's she met at the Mars Bar the night Darren DJed.

I approached them cautiously, all sorts of scenarios racing through my mind. What if he'd told her all about the netball court affair? What if Darren had talked to him about what we'd discussed at my house the night before and now he was telling Emma? Emma would think I'd betrayed her, that I'd been blabbing her personal business all around the school.

"Emma, what are you doing here?" I said, surprising them both so much that Gary jumped and poured Coke down his crisp white shirt. I was shaking inside but desperately trying to appear as calm as possible on the outside. "Oh, sorry, sorry. I didn't mean to make you jump."

Em got up and gave me a big hug. "I was walking past on my way home when Gary saw me and invited me in here for a coffee." She giggled and gave him a flirty look.

"Oh, right. I was just heading to the flat to see you, actually. Are you staying here long or what?" I was dying to get out of there and to be alone with Emma. I was praying that Gary wouldn't start talking about Claire Higgins or ask me if I'd gotten hurt in the fight. It was the talk of the school. Everyone had been whispering about it in corners all day. Sarah and I had spent every spare minute in our hideout, where I'd had a lot of explaining to do, especially after the extended assembly. Sarah had sat there with her jaw to the ground listening to everything I'd had to tell her. But even then I only told her about Claire Higgins on the netball court and being involved in a music workshop for an AIDS charity; I didn't go into anything about Em.

"Sit down. Get yourself a drink. What's the rush?" Emma said, grabbing my bag off my shoulder and moving up so that I could sit next to her.

"That party was mad on Friday night, wasn't it, Leyla? I

heard that Jimmy's parents came back early the next day and found four kids asleep in their bed and the dog pissed out of its head on gin that someone had poured into its water bowl for a laugh. I bet Jimmy has been grounded for life." Gary laughed and ordered another drink for himself.

It was agonizing. I was sure the next subject Gary would bring up was me and Claire Higgins. My stomach was in knots, but I knew I just had to go with the flow and not cause a fuss. "Yeah, he was freaking out right at the beginning of the party because a few glasses had been smashed," I said blithely. "Poor bloke. My parents know exactly what would happen to their precious home if they left me alone there for five minutes. I'd be sent to the electric chair if so much as a carpet thread was out of place." I hoped I was acting pretty much as usual.

We started telling each other different party anecdotes, but just as I started to relax a little I saw Claire Higgins emerge from behind the booth area at the back of the caff. I saw her stub out her cigarette and her entourage rise to follow her like sheep. My stomach lurched to my throat and I thought I was going to be sick there and then. As the blood rose to my cheeks, I knocked over the salt and pepper pots, spilling salt all over the table.

I wasn't scared of her but I really didn't want there to be any aggression while Emma was around. I'd managed to avoid Claire all day at school and knew that she'd have something to say to me at the first opportunity. I squirmed in my seat. I just wanted to protect Emma from any of this mess.

Even though I was keeping my head down, busying myself cleaning up the table, I could feel Claire coming closer. I realized that there would be more of a scene if she could see

I was trying to avoid her eye, so I tried to engage myself back into the conversation, acting as normal as possible. Emma and Gary seemed oblivious to how flustered I had become.

Claire approached our table and stood there with her hands on her hips. "My dad wants to know if you're going to cough up the deposit he put down for the school trip I've been banned from going on because you beat me up. He's round at your place as we speak, seeing if he can squeeze a few pennies out of your parents. I wouldn't like to be in your shoes when you get home tonight." She turned to the girls crowded round her, demanding their respect. They all laughed on cue and cast sneering looks in my direction.

I was enraged by her stinking attitude. Although I wanted to protect Emma, I had to wipe that smug look off Claire Higgins's face; she'd got away with too much already. I rummaged around in my purse for some coins and threw a fistful of coppers right at her. "There you go, Claire. Take it. You can have it all. I wish you were going to bloody Venice. I wish you'd drown in a sodding canal."

Georgio saw the kerfuffle and marched over, telling us to calm down or get out. "Don't worry I'm out of here," I announced. "Em, come on, let's go." Gobsmacked, Emma grabbed our bags and followed me out of the door, apologizing to Gary as we went. I stormed off down the street at top speed, forcing Emma to have to run to catch up with me.

"Leyla, what the hell is going on? Leyla, stop, I can't keep up," she said.

"I'll tell you everything back at the flat. I just want to get to the flat."

As I barged into the kitchen, I almost sent Aunty Jean flying. I marched past her and flung myself down on Emma's bed. To my mortification, I started to sob. Aunty Jean and Em soon followed, wondering what had got into me.

Aunty Jean knelt down at the side of the bed and asked me to tell her what was wrong. I hadn't planned on telling her anything. I thought I would just explain things to Em and take it from there, but instead I got all tearful and told them both everything, from how the subject of the workshop had come up with Darren in the first place to how my parents had been dragged into the whole affair. They sat quietly listening to everything I had to say, and when I'd finished Aunty Jean got up and stood at the window and didn't say anything for ages. Emma just cuddled up to me on the bed.

Eventually Aunty Jean turned round and told us that it was time she had a talk with my parents. "I don't want you getting into any more trouble. They need to know what's going on in Emma's life so that they can understand what's going on in yours, Leyla. I've been totally irresponsible in not telling them before now, just hoping that everything would go away and things would get back to normal after a while. Well, it's not *going* to go away, is it? And the longer we carry on hiding all of this, the worse it's going to get for everyone. They need to know."

I knew that she was right, but I was terrified of what my parents were going to say. "Leyla, I want you to stay here with Emma," Aunty Jean said firmly. "I'm going to go up to the house. Don't worry. I'll be back soon."

Emma and I stayed huddled on the bed, barely talking. We were together, and that was the most important thing. I felt totally drained by the past couple of days' events and was glad to have shared all of the stress with someone.

A couple of hours must have gone by when we heard

Aunty Jean let herself back into the flat. We both leapt to our feet and ran out to the kitchen. She didn't have to say anything, I could see from the look on her face that my parents hadn't taken the news well. She couldn't even raise her head to look at us.

Anger swelled up inside me. I felt like an inflated balloon that was just about to burst. How could they be so cruel? How could they be so ignorant and cruel? Emma is ill. She hasn't murdered or robbed anyone. She's just ill. Couldn't they understand that we'd had to lie because we knew that they'd react this way? I stood in the middle of the kitchen with my arms limp at my sides and couldn't find the energy to ask any questions. Emma went over to her mum and gave her a hug.

"Diane said that it was all my fault for not bringing Emma up properly," Aunty Jean explained. "That if I'd been a better mother and paid more attention to what she was getting up to she would never have gone sleeping with anyone in the first place." Emma gasped and covered her ears, sinking into the nearest chair. "She said that Emma was probably leading you astray as we spoke and that if she found out you had been as promiscuous as Emma she'd never let you out of her sight ever again." Aunty Jean started to sob uncontrollably. I was left speechless and shaking with fear and anger. "She wants you to go home immediately."

"I'm not going home. I can't go home to them. How can I go anywhere near them?" I spat out the words.

Emma stood up and put her arm around my shoulders. "Leyla, they're your parents; they just want to protect you. If anyone can talk some sense into them, it's you. Your mum has got such a chip on her shoulder about my mum and the way their whole family turned out that she's just lashing out. You know they don't get on. You'll be able to get through to her. You can tell her that I'm not some dirty slapper who deserves all I get. You can tell her that HIV isn't some filthy disease that you can catch from simply being in my company. You've got to be brave, Leyla. Things will come right in the end."

"I kept hoping all the way up there that they'd surprise me and be totally supportive and understanding, but deep down I knew what their reaction would be. This is more about me than you, love. You must remember that, darling." Aunty Jean put her arms out to Emma. "She doesn't wish you any harm, Em. She's a good woman really. She's just disappointed with the hand life has dealt her, and she sees me as part of that rotten pack of cards. I've let the family down in her eyes, and for Diane this is just more evidence of my irresponsible behavior. She doesn't mean you any harm, love."

I was shocked to hear Aunty Jean talk about my mum like that. I'd never thought about my mum actually being "disappointed" with life. I'd never thought of her as having any sort of hopes or dreams of her own. She was just my mum. I couldn't imagine her harboring any profound thoughts. She did the housework, looked after all of us, had her little routine, and seemed to exist comfortably in the home that she'd built up for us.

But if she was so disappointed with her lot, why did she keep pushing me in the same direction as her life had gone? Why did she want me to do the "sensible thing" of getting a decent job and settling down with a family in a nice house instead of pursuing my dream of becoming a drummer? Why was she so hell-bent on me and Sadie behaving respectably and properly all the time? She was always so worried about what the neighbors would think about our every move. Her life seemed to be stifled and restrained by her constant efforts to keep up a respectable front. It was a wonder she hadn't suffocated by now. "I just don't understand how you two are so different. Mum is so stuck in her ways. She's being really cruel. Why's she being like this? Why's she treating us like this?" I asked Aunty Jean.

"Leyla, there is so much you don't know that maybe you should. Your mum'll probably kill me for telling you, but you're old enough to know now." She took a deep breath before carrying on. "I fell pregnant with Emma when I was fifteen. I was a little girl really." Aunty Jean articulated each word carefully, like she was handling fragile pieces of glass. "It broke your grandma's heart, and she never really forgave me. She said that I'd brought shame on the family. Your mum was the eldest, so she had to be the responsible one and look after me; your grandma practically washed her hands of me. When Em was born I had no idea what to do with a baby, but your mum stuck by me all the way. As Sadie was nearly school age, your mum was supposed to go off to secretarial college, but she gave that up to look after me.

Emma was just two years old when I met your uncle Kevin. I fell head over heels in love, and he took me and Em in. I suppose I neglected your mum after that, because I had someone else to look after me. I must have hurt her terribly. The whole town was talking about me, so she felt she could never hold her head up high, and she'd lost her chance to go to college, since she'd just had you by that point as well. She's turned into a snob because of what happened and hates my guts because I never said thank you for all that she did for me. That's what all of this is about. She's seeing history repeat itself, in a way, and I deserve nothing less, according to her."

I was stunned. Everything was piecing together. I always wondered why Mum and Aunty Jean never got on and why Mum hated Uncle Kevin so much. It made sense now that Mum wanted me and Sadie to be normal and respectable and go about our lives keeping a low profile. She'd seen how life can knock you down when you're least expecting it. Perhaps she didn't want me to get my hopes up about leading a different sort of life, totally removed from the safe, humdrum routine she'd worked out for herself, because she was scared of the disappointment I might feel one day too.

I'd never ever thought of Mum in this way before. I'd never really looked beneath the surface. She was just my mum, who got on my nerves, who was on my back all the time, who kept everything ticking over in the house. I had no idea life had been so devastating for her.

"You all right, Leyla?" Emma was shoving a cup of tea under my nose. "Shocked to hear about my mum having me at fifteen, are you? It doesn't bother me. She's always been honest with me, and that's the most important thing. It was your mum who wanted it kept from you, because she thought it would set a bad example. No wonder she's freaked out about what's happened to me. She's just scared stiff for you. It'll be all right, Leyla. It's like my mum says—she's a good woman really."

"I'd better get back. I should talk to them, I suppose," I muttered.

"I told them all about the amazing work you're doing at the support center. I said it was a lifeline for Emma and that your music was helping a whole bunch of kids. They can't ignore all of that, Leyla. You're a good kid, and they know it," Aunty Jean said soothingly.

When I got home Mum and Dad were sat in the living room in silence with the television turned off. The television was never off in our house. I looked at Mum sat there on the sofa, with her hands folded neatly on her lap, the veins on her neck taut and strained, and I suddenly felt that the new knowledge and insight I had was too much for me to bear. It was easy when she had been just Mum, with no major emotions or traumas or any sort of private life outside of this home, but now it was much more complex and there was so much to take into consideration. I felt as though I'd just taken a huge leap forward in this whole growing-up malarkey. My relationship with Mum would never be the same again—and perhaps that wasn't such a bad thing.

But my thoughts soon turned to Emma, and I knew I had to make them understand what she was going through and what, as a result, I was going through as well. There was no point beating about the bush. I had to be frank and honest all the way.

I stood in front of them in the middle of the living room. "So you know about Emma?"

"Yes, and if we find out you've been as loose as—" Mum began to shriek, but Dad stopped her mid-flow and adopted a more gentle, caring approach.

"Listen, love, we're concerned about you, we're—" he began.

"Stop. Just stop." It was my turn to do the talking. I had so much to say, I didn't know where to start. "Emma has got HIV. She needs love and support from her family more than anything in the world. She didn't want this to happen to her. HIV is totally indiscriminate; it doesn't choose bad people over good people. It can happen to anyone who isn't careful.

I've learnt a lesson about safe sex the hardest way anyone ever could—by seeing Emma end up like this. She doesn't deserve to be treated like an outcast. She's our flesh and blood; she needs us.

"I'm scared as well, you know. I feel totally helpless half the time, but the one thing I realized I could do for her was help out at the support center, drumming. So don't be angry with me—I've just been helping the only way I know how. And you don't need to be worried about me. I'm perfectly safe. I'm not going to catch HIV from anyone. I'm just trying to help Emma."

My words hung heavily in the air. No one knew what to say next, and I realized that perhaps now wasn't the time to do any more talking. I got up and went to bed.

TWELVE

THE FOLLOWING SATURDAY I GOT READY TO GO TO THE support center with Emma as usual. The atmosphere in the house all week had been subdued, but not hostile. Nobody had spoken about Emma or Aunty Jean, and I had decided to leave Mum and Dad to think. I couldn't expect miracles from them in a few days, and as long as they weren't coming out with a load of bullshit I was happy for them to just leave me to get on with things for a while. But I'd also decided that I was going to be completely open about everything to do with Emma and my involvement in her life. I wasn't going to hide anything anymore.

Just before I left the house, I popped my head around the kitchen door. "I'm off to the support center with Emma. See you later." I didn't wait for a reply.

On the way there, Emma told me that she'd phoned the

center to tell them about the incident with Claire Higgins and how it was her brother who worked at the music college who had been talking about the group in school. Lucinda and Graham decided to move the music workshop back to the center to ensure everyone's security. The music college lent them some equipment—a drum kit, a keyboard, an electric guitar, a sequencer, and some mikes—so that the workshops could carry on.

The minute I walked in the door, Shula mobbed me to show off some new techniques she'd been practicing on the drums. Ellie and Emma were still as captivated as ever by Justine and hung on her every word. They were following her example and doing some warm-up scales and vocal exercises. Glen was teaching Rafi how to tune a guitar. Benjamin and Dotun were recording some samples onto a four-track Dave had brought in and mixing down some keyboard parts onto a recording Glen had done of some ideas for a melody. They were definitely the technical bods of the group, while Emma and Ellie liked to think of themselves as the greatest divas of all time. Shula and Rafi were dedicated to learning to play an instrument and were completely enthralled with the drums and the guitar.

It was all coming together nicely. Everyone had found their particular niche within the group. Graham came in to talk to us later in the day about fund-raising. The center was struggling financially and risked being closed down if more funds weren't found soon. Money from trustees and anonymous benefactors was running dry, and the center had reached crisis point. The adults were doing a sponsored walk and an aerobics-athon, and Graham wanted to know if we had any fund-raising ideas ourselves and would be willing to participate in any events. We spent at least an hour firing ideas at one another—bike rides, dance-athons, read-athons, sponsored swims, club nights—most of which everyone had done before and were bored of. Nobody seemed particularly keen, and it wasn't looking good.

Then the idea came to me as I looked around the room full of music equipment. Everyone was obviously really enthusiastic about the music workshop, so I thought that we could make a CD and sell it to raise money. I hesitantly put the idea to the group.

"Why don't we do something with our music," I suggested. "We could make a CD, like a charity record, and sell it. Nobody would have to be named on the CD. It could all be completely anonymous and just have the name of the support center on it, with all proceeds going to this worthy cause. It's easy to get CDs done these days."

My suggestion was greeted with blank faces. Nobody was interested.

"You won't catch me making some naff save-the-world ballad to get everyone blubbing into their hankies," Rafi piped up, twisting his baseball cap round and round his head.

Shula was next. "We're not good enough anyway. I've only just figured out where the bass drum is on that kit. I couldn't play on a *record*."

Graham suggested we go home and think some more about fund-raising ideas and get back to him after Christmas, which was the following week. We all left, hardly in the festive mood, convinced that the center was going to close down, and I went away feeling like a fool for suggesting such an unpopular idea as making a CD.

The Saturday after New Year the center was closed for an

emergency staff meeting about finances. I went round to Darren's house. He'd just passed his guitar exams and his mum had bought him an eight-track for Christmas and to celebrate his exam results. We thought we'd have a go at recording some stuff.

Mrs. Mitchell answered the door. "Hello, dear. Come on in. Don't look at me, though, I'm not wearing a scrap of makeup. I've just been for a facial and haven't had time to put my face back on. Did you want a drink or anything? Oh, I've got these lovely sachets of ninety percent fat-free hot chocolate that I had from my slimming club last week. Just what you need on a day like today."

She hadn't given me a chance to say no, so I followed her into the kitchen.

"Darren's upstairs having a snooze, I think," she continued. "He was in late again last night. DJing till all hours." She leant against the kitchen table as she waited for the kettle to boil. "I worry about him. God knows what you youngsters get up to in those clubs. I read the newspapers. He'll be hooked on that ecstasy before he knows it."

I didn't know where to put myself. I didn't want to be having this conversation with her. I just nodded and made the right noises while willing the kettle to boil faster.

"Did you go to that Jimmy's party just before Christmas?" she asked suddenly.

"Umm, yes," I answered reluctantly, not sure if it was a trick question.

"I heard they had the police round there at six in the morning with sniffer dogs. They did a big drugs raid. Found a kilo of cocaine and God knows what else."

"Mum, you are exaggerating so badly." Darren was stood

in the doorway. I hadn't heard him come downstairs. "The police went round there because the neighbors complained about the music. They didn't find any drugs whatsoever. What is your problem?"

"My problem is you going out till all hours and not getting any sleep. You're not telling me you stay awake on a few cups of coffee."

"Mum, I'm eighteen years old. I'm young. Get off my back." He took my hand and led me upstairs, leaving his mum to rant on alone. "She doesn't half go on," Darren moaned once we were out of the kitchen.

"Well, she still buys you things like your eight-track. She's worried about you, but at least she supports you. My mum and dad would sell my drum kit in a carboot sale if they had half the chance."

We spent the day holed up in his room recording guitar riffs and drum sequences from his drum machine onto his eight-track, with bits of our favorite records mixed in. The end result of our day's work was a tapeful of disjointed pieces of music that we were both convinced would be auctioned off for a fortune once we became musical legends.

Before I went home I popped in to see how Emma was doing. It was the first Saturday in ages that she hadn't been to the support center and she'd been out shopping with her mum.

"How was your day then, Em? Was it nice to be doing what you'd normally do on a Saturday instead of being at the center?" I asked her.

"Yeah, we had a good day, but to be honest I did miss the group. I've just got stuck into that singing lark. And I've got quite close to Shula and Ellie. I keep wondering how Shula's coping with her mum and if Ellie's come any closer to telling her boyfriend. And do you reckon the center will find some funds?"

"I hope so. It'd be awful if they closed down."

"I'm dead worried about it. I know I'm lucky to have you and Mum; some people don't have anyone outside of Positive Living they can turn to. But it's different with everyone at the center. I don't feel so alone when I go there. I walk in the door and know that everyone there is in the same boat as me so I don't have to feel so scared. It's like I've got two identities or something: one identity at college and another when I'm at the center. I can just chill out when I'm there. I can be myself, talk about HIV openly if I want to, and I don't have to worry about what people will say when I'm taking my tablets. I don't think I could handle it if it had to close down."

"We've got to get some dosh from somewhere. I felt such a knob when I suggested that CD idea, though."

"No way, I think it's a good idea. I reckon we should do it. I felt too intimidated to say anything the other week because no one else was interested and I didn't want to look as though I was being all bigheaded thinking that I was good enough to make a record, but I'll bring it up again next week. We've got to try *something*."

"Well, I've been round at Darren's making this tape all day. We've had a right laugh. But perhaps I could take it to the group next week to give them some idea of what we could do." I played Emma the tape and she loved what we'd done, even declaring it a work of genius, which was a little over the top, but it made her more determined than ever to get the CD idea off the ground.

Emma stuck to her word, and the next Saturday she proposed my idea of putting a CD together. "There'll be loads of practicalities to work out, but if we can get three good songs together to start with and then decide how and where it's going to be recorded, at least we'll have got the ball rolling. What's the alternative—another sponsored walk! We'd be doing something that all of our hearts are in already. Justine and Leyla and the others will help us all the way."

Everyone sat and thought about it while I crossed my fingers and prayed that they would come to their senses.

"I've got some lyrics that I wrote here," Ellie said warily. "Perhaps we could use them on one of the songs."

"So do you want to do it then?" Emma asked Ellie and the rest of the group.

"I'm not sitting round any campfire with an acoustic guitar writing protest songs," Rafi voiced.

"I'm not doing any of that 'bitch, whore, pussy' gangsta rap that you listen to, either," Shula responded, sucking her teeth.

"Does this mean you're up for it or not? Put your hand in the air if you want to make a CD," Emma persisted.

Ellie, Emma, Glen, Dave, Justine, Shula, and me raised our hands without hesitation. Benjamin and Dotun followed. Rafi eventually took off his cap and waved it above his head to show that he was in.

"Move over, Justine: There's a new kid on the block," Ellie joked, puffing out her chest.

"Who says *you're* taking vocals? I've got you penciled in for the tambourine," Justine teased.

Graham reminded us that the center would probably have closed down by the time we got our acts together to make some music, let alone raise any funds out of it. He suggested that we set a realistic schedule and aim to have three songs recorded by March, which was in two months' time.

When the taxi drove into Bury that evening, Emma asked the driver if he would go straight up to my estate, Beech Glen, instead of dropping her off at the flat.

"Why aren't you getting out first?" I demanded.

"I'm coming to see your parents."

"Why?" I asked, aghast.

"Well, they can't avoid me for the rest of their lives; they've got to see me at some point. And besides, Mum has been so cut up since their conversation I thought I could perhaps talk some sense into them, make them see what they're doing to this family. Mum hasn't got anyone. She should at least be able to turn to her own sister."

"Yes, but you heard what your mum was saying about getting pregnant with you and then Uncle Kevin coming along. I don't think it's as easy as all that, Em. You might make things worse."

"Let's face it, Leyla—things can't *get* much worse."

I had a really rotten feeling about her impromptu visit. Emma didn't know Mum like I did, and I knew this could backfire pretty badly. But there was no stopping Emma; she was determined to have her say.

I went on ahead into the living room while Emma took off her shoes and coat in the hall. Mum and Dad didn't even bother to acknowledge me, but when Emma walked in and said hello they both looked as though they'd seen a ghost. Though you could have cut the atmosphere with a knife, Dad tried to act normal. "Hello, Emma. We haven't seen you round here for ages." Mum was either speechless or busy preparing a speech, I couldn't quite figure out which.

"We've just got back from the music group. We're going to

put out a CD and try to sell it to raise some funds. I'll be drumming on it. So you'll be able to go out and buy a CD that your daughter has helped make." I thought they'd be glad to hear that something productive was coming out of my Saturdays away from the fold.

"Leyla's a star, you know," Emma joined in. "She's been amazing to me and my mum, and an inspiration to the group." I could see that Emma was shaking a little. We were still stood up looking awkward and vulnerable. I motioned her to sit down on the sofa with me.

"How is your mum?" Dad asked innocently, not seeming to realize what a loaded question it was. I expected sparks to fly, bombs to explode, heads to roll, and felt I should warn Mum and Dad to run for cover. Instead Emma sat up straight and calmly answered him.

"She's in a terrible state, actually. She's not eating properly, she's taken days off work—which she can't afford—she hasn't had a full night's sleep in weeks. She's a bag of nerves."

"Oh, I didn't . . . I didn't realize . . . ," Dad mumbled.

I'm not usually lost for words when it comes to speaking my mind in front of my parents, but I wasn't quite sure how to handle this particular situation. I wished Mum would say something so that at least things would be out in the open.

"She's pretty upset about what happened round here the other week," Emma continued bravely. "She's got no one to talk to about what's happening in our lives. She needs you, Aunty Diane. Leyla's been a rock for both of us, but Mum needs as much support as possible if we're going to get through this."

Mum just stared at us both, not saying a word. I couldn't begin to read her expression.

"Aunty Diane, please talk to her. She just needs to know you're there—"

Mum didn't give Emma the chance to finish her sentence. She got up and walked out of the room, shutting the door carefully and deliberately behind her. We followed the sound of her footsteps upstairs and into the bedroom. The bed creaked as she sat down and the low tones of a Radio 4 presenter drifted downstairs.

"So, will you make any money out of this CD then?" Dad queried.

"Oh shut up, Dad."

THIRTEEN

I COULDN'T QUITE BELIEVE IT. EMMA TOLD ME THE news at Georgio's after school, but I was too upset to really take it all in. Aunty Jean had decided to move down to London, and to take Emma with her, of course. She wanted a fresh start for them both. She'd threatened to do it before Christmas, but Emma had managed to convince her to stay. There was no stopping her this time, however. They would have better access to medical treatments and experts in HIV down there. Aunty Jean had a few friends who she reckoned could get her a better job so that she could give Emma a higher standard of living and afford to see her through university. She'd also started to worry that rumors about Em would get out soon and wanted to protect her before anything nasty happened. Aunty Jean knew how cruel people could be. She couldn't bear to see it happen to Em.

My mum hadn't spoken to either Aunty Jean or Emma since she'd found out. For that matter, Mum and Dad hadn't really spoken to me about it either, despite my best efforts. They never tried to stop me from going to the center, but they wouldn't talk about it. They just clammed up on the issue entirely. I'm pretty sure they didn't know what to say or do, so they kept their mouths shut and their heads down.

I left leaflets about HIV and AIDS around the house, only to find them in the bin one day. I tried talking to them when we were all sat watching telly together, but they blanked it out. They didn't want to know. I saw Mum crying one afternoon, sat at the kitchen table with a pen in her hand. I made her jump when I walked in, and she shuffled things away on the table and brushed her tears off as her just feeling tired and emotional.

I wasn't sure if it was a coincidence, but since it was Emma's seventeenth birthday I wondered if she was trying to write a card. However, Emma didn't receive anything from her, for the first year ever. Mum usually sends a card with a twenty-pound note inside, but not this year. Aunty Jean came round the house again to try and talk to them, but Mum slammed the door in her face. I refused to go home for a whole weekend after that and stayed down at the flat until Aunty Jean forced me to go back.

Sadie hasn't got a clue what's going on. Mum and Dad haven't told her anything, which is frustrating the hell out of her. Her and Anthony overheard a woman calling Aunty Jean a slag down at the pub one night. When she said, "Like mother, like daughter," Sadie saw red and punched her. Mum was mortified, naturally. She couldn't believe Sadie had shown the family up so badly and forbade her from showing her face at the Bull and Gate ever again. But Mum still didn't tell Sadie about Em. She just carried on as normal, sticking to her routines, never letting her stony-faced façade slip.

If there was one thing I'd learnt, it was that families could be really stubborn and stupid. You'd think that your own flesh and blood would stand by you through all of life's ups and downs. But families can bear grudges for the whole of their lives, refusing to forgive and forget.

Mum had dug her feet in so firmly I wondered if she'd ever be able to make any positive move forward. I could have screamed; it was so absurd, and so ugly. All Mum had to do was show some sign of compassion or support for Emma and Aunty Jean and they wouldn't have to move to the other end of the country to start a new life. I knew that Mum wasn't the only factor in Aunty Jean's decision to move, but her attitude wasn't exactly encouraging my aunt and cousin to stick around, either.

Emma had become my soul mate. I couldn't imagine her not being around. She trusted me; she leant on me, I was always there for her, and I relied on her just as much. I wondered if Aunty Jean had thought about the consequences of splitting us up. I knew that it wasn't the other side of the world, but if something happened to her I'd want to be close enough to be by her side at a moment's notice. It was all so unfair and inconsiderate.

We'd only just got things together musicwise for the CD as well. We'd written two songs and were halfway through the third. Emma was doing the lead vocals for the first track, and it was sounding brilliant. She was so proud of what she'd done it was inconceivable that she wouldn't be around to see the whole thing through to completion.

I wondered if I would still be allowed to attend the center if Emma was no longer there. She was the only reason I'd gone there in the first place, but as Lucinda and Graham pointed out, I was affected by HIV as well and needed the support that the group offered. I'd made so many new friends and given up so much time and energy to the music workshop it felt like just as much my space as Emma's.

Aunty Jean wanted to leave during half term, at the end of February, so that Emma wouldn't have to miss too much school. It simply wouldn't sink in that she wasn't going to be down the road in the flat or sat drinking coffee in Georgio's or that I wouldn't bump into her at a club or a party.

These bloody grown-ups had got a lot to answer for.

"You've got a lot to answer for," I screamed from my bedroom, banging my feet on the floor. "Do you hear me? You've got a lot to answer for."

Silence. They didn't dare stir. The thought of the awful silence that lurked in every corner of our lives made my blood boil.

FOURTEEN

EMMA HAD BEEN LIVING IN LONDON A MONTH. SHE'D started a new college, Aunty Jean had got herself a job working as a PA in a law firm, and they seemed to have settled in quite well. Emma and I phoned each other every other night and talked for at least an hour. She was doing fine. She'd got to know a few people at her new college and her mum was a lot happier, so that was something at least.

I missed her like mad, but I'd been keeping myself busy with the music group and seemed to spend every spare moment working on the CD project, so I hadn't had much time to mope around. We'd finished writing all three songs and had sent Emma tapes each week so that she could still be a part of it. I'd been trying to get a CD producer interested in helping us out for weeks, but no one was interested. Everyone was too busy, too booked up, too bloody lazy.

It was Friday night, and I was compiling a letter to send out to some well-known producers to ask them—beg them—for their time and help. If we found a producer, the next step would be to find a recording studio. It was so expensive, though, that I didn't know if we'd ever be able to afford it. There was the cost of a producer, a technician, equipment hire, hire of the studio itself. Nobody seemed to want to give us anything for free. But we were all determined to see the songs pressed to CD, even if it didn't make any money. We'd worked too hard to give up.

I hadn't seen Darren for a few days, but he'd promised to call tonight. He was DJing at a club in town and he thought he could get me on the guest list. We hadn't been on a big night out in weeks. I'd been neglecting Sarah a bit as well since I'd got so involved with the music workshop, and I thought it would be a good opportunity to go out with her, if she hadn't already found a whole new bunch of mates to hang out with on Friday nights.

Darren called to say that he'd put me and Sarah on the guestie, so I got on the phone to her straightaway. "Sarah, what are you doing tonight?"

"Hmm, let's see, hold on a minute, let me just get the TV guide. Okay, well, at eight o'clock there's *Brookie*—oh, and before that *Coronation Street*. I might fit in a bit of revision—we do have exams this year, you know—then there's *Friends, South Park,* and *Frasier.* Why?"

"I was wondering if I could tear you away to come out clubbing with me?"

"Sorry, this is a really bad line." I could hear Sarah banging the phone against the hall table a few times. "It must be a crossed line. I thought I just heard someone ask me if I wanted to go out clubbing tonight."

"Okay, sarky pants. So I haven't been out clubbing for all of . . . oh, let's see—three weeks. It's not a crime, you know."

"A lot can happen in three weeks in the world of fashion and music, Leyla. There's probably been a totally new musical phenomenon sweeping the nation's dance floors since we were last out. There'll be a whole new range of club gear that people are wearing and we'll turn up in our bindis and stacked sneakers looking like a couple of out-of-touch parents."

"You are mad. You're mad. You've lost it; I'm calling the men in white coats to come and get you. I'll give you one last chance. Do you want to come out with your best mate tonight or not?"

"Where are we going?"

"Does that mean you're coming?"

"Where are we going?"

"Darren's DJing at the Music Box on Oxford Road. He's put us on the guest list. There'll be a gang of people from school there. Are you up for it or not?"

"Yeah, okay then. It's got to beat a night in with my mum and her mate Jesus. But don't blame me if we don't know the right moves on the dance floor or if we're turned away at the door for looking way too uncool."

"I'll be at your house by eight thirty, you nutter."

When we got there, Darren was milling around at the entrance to the club like he owned the place. He knew practically everyone who went in through the doors. My stomach flipped when I saw him, and I realized how much I'd missed him. I was so happy to be out with him and Sarah that I promised myself not to neglect either of them again. I'd been so wrapped up in the music project and the whole family situation I'd forgotten I had such amazing friends, and that they meant the world to me.

All three of us walked downstairs to the dark underground venue, then dropped into an entrance area that you had to go through before you got to the main room. The toilets were down there as well and they'd already flooded, so we had to tread carefully through half an inch of water. Camouflage netting was draped around the walls and ceiling, with hundreds of Barbie and Ken dolls in compromising positions entwined in it. Darren opened the door for us into the main room. We could barely see our hands in front of our faces for all the dry ice. A row of glitter-covered shop mannequins with cowboy hats on their heads propped up the bar, indicating the place where we could get a drink. Cheap, watered-down spirits were going for a quid a shot. Popper bottles littered the floor. Drum 'n' bass boomed from amps stacked to the ceiling. A sweaty mass of seminaked bodies throbbed together on the dance floor.

It was everything that Darren's mother feared. It was her worst nightmare come true. It was bliss.

Darren DJed between eleven and twelve thirty, and when he finally reemerged from behind his stack of records I managed to get him to myself. We sneaked off into a dimly lit corner and pounced on each other. I didn't want to stop kissing him. I felt as though I had to make up for lost time, but we eventually came up for air and actually talked.

"So what have you been up to this week?" I asked.

"It's been quite an exciting week, actually. The other night I was round at a friend's house whose older brother is in this band who've just signed a singles deal with that Manchester label, Faith and Hope. They're going into the studio next week, and they want an extra lead guitar on one of the tracks, so they've asked me if I'd like to do it. I hadn't even heard the song until Wednesday, but I've been working on it and it's going to be good. I'm dead excited."

"Wow, that's so cool, you lucky bugger. I wish *we* could get a producer and a studio. Everyone and everywhere is so expensive. You'd think they'd do it for free for charity, but no scumbag will touch us. We've worked so hard on these songs; I don't want to see them go to waste."

"Well, I might make some contacts who would be willing to help you out. I'll keep my eyes open for you. Of course, I'll have to hear your stuff first before I go raving about it."

"Okay, come round the house tomorrow and I'll play you our tape. I guarantee you'll be playing it in here next time you're spinning those choons."

The following Wednesday at school, Sarah and I were sat in our secret place at lunchtime when Darren burst in, looking cockier than ever.

"Oh my God, have I got a surprise for you," he said, picking me up off the floor and swinging me around.

"Don't tell me. Noel Gallagher personally came round to your house and asked you to play on the next Oasis album," Sarah said. She was deeply suspicious of Darren's continuing success in everything he put his hand to, and in her usual cynical way was convinced the bubble had to burst soon.

"No, but he might well be knocking on Leyla's door after he's heard the CD she'll be putting out in a matter of weeks." Darren grinned.

"What are you talking about? We haven't even got a recording studio."

"You have now," he said, kissing me. "On Monday I went out with that band I was telling you about and met their producer. I told him all about the support group and how you had helped set up a music workshop there and were trying to put out a CD to raise funds for the center. He couldn't believe that nobody had wanted to help you. He owns his own studio on Great Ancoats Street, and told me to pop by with you sometime this week. He said he'd be willing to give you free studio space and equipment to use and that he'd produce it for you—all for free."

I was speechless. Even Sarah was stunned—so stunned that she couldn't manage to pull a sarcastic comment out of her hat. I just hugged and hugged and hugged Darren until he eventually asked me to say something.

"What can I say? I'm blown away."

"'Thanks' would be a start." Sarah nudged me.

"Oh, sorry. Thank you, thank you. It's brilliant news. It's fantastic. When can we go in? Oh God, I don't think we're ready. Everyone's going to be so happy. I've got to go and phone the center. We need to call an emergency session. What if he changes his mind?"

"He won't change his mind. He's cool. Name the date and it's all yours."

FIFTEEN

WE FINALLY GOT THE CD RECORDED, THANKS TO
Darren and his mate. It all happened pretty quickly—we went
into the studio a couple of weekends and got it all done in two
days. Everyone worked brilliantly together, and Emma surprised us all by turning up at the studio at the very last
minute, so she managed to get her voice on the record she'd
worked so hard for. She couldn't stay away—if there was ever
any hint of her getting her fifteen minutes of fame, then
Emma was always going to be there.

The trouble was, I'd been trying to contact her for a
couple of days to tell her that we'd had fifty CDs pressed up
and sent out to radio stations and anyone else influential we
could think of, and there was no answer at her new house.
I knew how excited she'd be, if only I could get ahold of
her. I was sure she would have told me if she was going

away anywhere. I'd tried phoning Aunty Jean at work, but they said she'd been off sick for a few days. What if something had happened to her? Why hadn't Aunty Jean been in touch? Normally she would have called me. I knew that something had to be wrong.

SIXTEEN

I WAS LYING STAR-SHAPED ON MY BED IN THE POKY box bedroom of our semidetached house on a Wednesday night staring at the four walls hemming me in, longing for some help, some courage, when I was jolted out of my deep thoughts by the sound of Mr. Davies rummaging next door. It wasn't the usual day for his pipe, so I sat up and peered through the window and waited for him to appear. But I saw Mrs. Davies out in the garden instead.

She had a great big shovel in her hand. I watched open-mouthed as she dug a hole in the middle of Mr. Davies's vegetable patch and ceremoniously threw his pipe into the grave she'd made for it. I found myself clapping as she covered the hole back up with dirt. When she'd finished, she looked up at me in the window and took a bow.

Mrs. Davies had given me all the courage I needed. Her

little ceremony made me realize that you didn't have to put up with things the way they were just because they'd always been that way; not if you didn't want to. It was good to take action sometimes.

I'd received a letter from Aunty Jean that morning telling me that Emma had been in hospital for the past four days. She'd caught the flu, and because she'd been so run-down with all of the stress of moving to London and everything, her body couldn't fight it off like normal and she was put on a ventilator for a chronic chest infection.

I'd decided to go and see her, but I was scared. Scared of not being able to cope with her being ill, scared of how Aunty Jean was going to be feeling, scared of Emma dying. But I knew I had to go and see her.

I hadn't told Mum and Dad, but I was going no matter what they said. Aunty Jean had been in that hospital by Em's bedside the whole time, with no one to help out or to take turns sitting with Em. She hadn't even had the energy or the will to get to a phone and call me to let me know what had happened for fear of my mum answering and rejecting her yet again. That's why she'd written the letter. It was midweek and I had exams coming up, but I needed to see them. I was frantic with worry. I'd found out train times from Manchester Piccadilly and had managed to speak to Aunty Jean at the hospital just after the letter arrived. She said she'd pick me up at Euston and take me to see Em. I packed a little rucksack. Now I just had to get past my parents.

Downstairs, Mum and Dad were watching the National Lottery show and weren't too happy when I plonked myself in front of the telly.

"Shift yourself, we could be millionaires any moment and

we'd miss it," Dad shouted, clutching his Lottery ticket and pushing me out of the way.

"Where are you going with that bag?" Mum said curiously.

"I'm going to London to see Emma."

"You're not," Mum said, shifting from her slouched position to an upright one on the edge of the sofa. "Tell her, Jeremy—she's not going to London on her own. It's Wednesday night. She's got school tomorrow and important exams coming up." Mum jabbed Dad in the ribs.

Dad was engrossed in the Lottery and was striking off numbers on his ticket with an exaggerated sweep of his pen. "Fifteen. Yes. Thirty-two. Yes. Oh my God, this is it, I can feel it in my water. Forty-seven. Yes. Diane, we're going to be rich!" Dad was on his feet, his face inches away from the TV screen, punching the air with a jubilant fist each time he got a number.

Meanwhile, Mum and I locked horns and prepared for battle. We were equally stubborn, and it was going to take a hell of a lot for either of us to back down. "Six. *Yes.* I'm going to be sick. We've got four numbers. Two to go. I don't believe it." Dad grabbed hold of Mum's waist and picked her up so that her size-five slippered feet were two inches off the floor. Neither of us could carry on ignoring what my dad was getting so excited about.

With our eyes and mouths wide open, all three of us turned to the screen and waited as the final numbers appeared. I could buy a new drum kit, I thought. I could buy a whole recording studio, or even a record company. I could buy Emma the best treatment in the world. There was total silence in the living room as the balls rolled around the tombola, like the deafening silence a car crash victim experiences split seconds before impact.

When the next two balls rolled into place, it was like a car crash *had* taken place, in the middle of our living room. Dad dropped Mum as suddenly as he'd picked her up and let out an enormous groan of disappointment before slumping back down onto the sofa, his head in his hands.

"Twenty-bloody-four. Twenty-four and a sixteen and we'd have been dining on caviar and champagne for the rest of our lives. We were so close. So close." He threw the doomed ticket onto the floor and hid behind a crumpled newspaper to sulk.

I picked up the rucksack I'd dropped in the excitement and made my way to the door. "I'm going to see Em, Mum, and you can't stop me. She's ill. She's in hospital. Aunty Jean sent me this letter. She's picking me up at the station in London, and I'll be fine." I handed her the letter, but she let it flutter to the floor as she stared indignantly at me. I turned my back and headed out onto the street.

It was dark outside, and pouring down with rain, but at least it diluted my tears as I stumbled toward the bus stop to get a bus to the train station. The tears were for Emma, for me, and for Mum—especially for Mum. I knew that she wanted to throw up her arms and break down in grief, but history stopped her in her tracks. Too much time had passed; she'd grown too stubborn and too proud to climb down from her position of superiority. She'd built an icy shield all around her, one I wanted to smash down with a sledgehammer. Too scared to try and bring down the protective shield herself, she'd decided a long time ago that it was easier to stay hidden behind it. But I knew she loved Aunty Jean and loved Emma like she was her own daughter. So I cried for Mum, too.

I was sat at the bus stop trying to control my sobbing—it

was causing passersby to stop and stare—when I heard a car screech to a halt right in front of me. Prepared to defend myself against some weirdo curb-crawler, I sat up straight and attempted to gather my wits. Then I saw that it was in fact Mum stepping out from behind the wheel. I couldn't bear another fight; I didn't have the energy. I wished she would just leave me alone.

"Come on, love, get in the car," she said, picking the bag up from my lap and holding out her hand.

I stayed where I was and, between sobs, managed to protest, "I'm not coming home, Mum. I need to see Emma."

Mum leant against the bus shelter, her thin jumper sticking to her body as the rain soaked through it. I noticed she still had her slippers on. She took a long, deep breath and said, "We're *going* to see Emma. We're going together. Come on, love." She put her arms around my shoulders and I let myself be led to the car, dragging my feet, my head hung low.

I was drenched from the rain, and overwhelmingly tired. I hadn't slept properly for nights with worrying about Emma, not knowing where she was. And it was suddenly as though all of the stress and worry of the past seven months since Emma told me that she was HIV positive had finally caught up with me in that single moment. I couldn't muster up a scrap of energy to ask my mum any questions. Why the change of heart? What did this mean for the future? All I cared about was that I was being taken to see Em. I just needed to see Em.

We drove in silence, watching the English countryside roll by in the darkness, both of us lost in our own grief and sadness. I thought about everything that had happened in the past seven months. It had been one long roller-coaster ride, and there had been plenty of times when I'd wanted to get off. But Emma was strapped in beside me, and there was no way I could leave her to face all those peaks and troughs and the scary upside-down bits all on her own.

Besides, you never knew where all those twists and turns were going to lead. I took a look at that cosmic shopping list of mine the other day and decided to make a few changes. I've changed wish number four, which I now regret writing all those months ago. "I want a good drama in my life" has been axed; "I want a good life in my drama" is my new wish. A good life for Emma, for Aunty Jean, for Mum, and for me.

Mum reached to turn on the radio as we hit the motorway. It was the usual conveyor belt pap, interspersed with criminally boring DJ banter. I kicked off my wet shoes, put my feet up on the dashboard, leant my head back, closed my eyes, and eventually fell into a light sleep—a sleep that I needed like a starving person needs food. But just as the stresses and strains temporarily left my mind, familiar music crept into my dreams. It swam around my head until I woke suddenly realizing that one of our songs was being played on the radio. Mum was tapping her hand on the wheel and humming along to our song. My drumbeats echoed around the car and throbbed inside my head like a fast, heavy pulse. They were actually playing our song. Emma's voice crept out from behind the guitars and whispered Ellie's poignant lyrics:

> You can't run away, it's here to stay.
> The die is cast and you won't be the last,
> But the beat goes on . . .

RESOURCES

Teen HIV/AIDS Resources

Hotlines

National Teen AIDS Prevention Hotline
1-800-234-TEEN
Monday–Friday, 1:00 P.M.–8:00 P.M.

National Teen AIDS Hotline
1-800-440-TEEN
Friday–Sunday, 6:00 P.M.–12:00 A.M.

Center for Disease Control Hotline
1-800-277-8922
24 hours/day, 7 days/week

Web Sites

I Wanna Know
www.iwannaknow.org
Teen-geared Web site

Planned Parenthood
www.plannedparenthood.org/sti/aidsquestions.html
Comprehensive, straightforward information

American Foundation for AIDS Research
www.thebody.com/amfar/youth_questions.html
Teen-friendly Web site

YouthHIV.org
www.youthHIV.org
Community site for HIV positive teens, including great
resources for safer sex

Teen Wire
www.teenwire.org
Colorful site aimed at tweens. Offers information on
sexuality, sexually transmitted infections, and puberty.

Advocates for Youth
www.advocatesforyouth.org
Extensive network of HIV/AIDS information and great
resources for sexual health activism programs

Ambiente Joven
www.ambientejoven.org
Spanish Web site for teens, providing plenty of information

Go Ask Alice
www.goaskalice.columbia.edu
Maintained by Columbia University, this helpful site covers
just about everything.

What You Do
www.whatudo.org
Well-designed site with a wide range of HIV/AIDS-related
information

Books

Alexander, Ruth Bell. *Changing Bodies, Changing Lives*
(Crown, 1998).

Basso, Michael. *The Underground Guide to Teenage Sexuality*
(Fairview Press, 1997).

Drill, Esther, Rebecca Odes, and Heather McDonald. *Deal
with It!: A Whole New Approach to Your Body, Brain, and Life as
a gURL* (Simon & Schuster, Pocket Books, 1999).